HOMOEOPATHY
THE FAMILY HANDBOOK

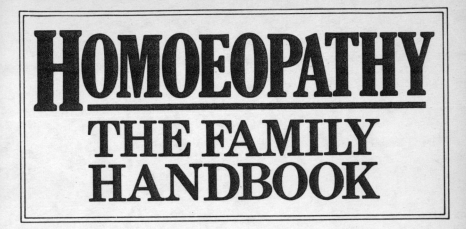

HOMOEOPATHY
THE FAMILY HANDBOOK

*An easily
understood guide
to the selection and use
of homoeopathic
medicines*

Recommended by
THE BRITISH HOMOEOPATHIC ASSOCIATION

Thorsons
An Imprint of HarperCollinsPublishers

Thorsons
An Imprint of HarperCollins*Publishers*
77-85 Fulham Palace Road,
Hammersmith, London W6 8JB

First published by Unwin Paperbacks, an imprint of
Unwin Hyman Limited 1987
Published by Thorsons 1992
1 3 5 7 9 10 8 6 4 2

© Wigmore Publication 1987, 1992

A catalogue record for this book
is available from the British Library

ISBN 0 7225 2721 7

Printed in Great Britain by
HarperCollinsManufacturing Glasgow

Acknowledgments

The publishers acknowledge the invaluable assistance provided by Mr J C Pert MRPharmS FSAO, Associate Member of the Faculty of Homoeopathy and various members of the Faculty of Homoeopathy in the preparation of this book.

Finally, but by no means least, they wish to thank Charlotte Reynolds for her untiring work without which the Handbook would never have appeared in its present form.

Contents

Introduction

This handbook has two objectives.

Its main aim is to provide a clear and easily understood introduction to Homoeopathy. It is not intended to deal with the subject in depth but to provide the newcomer with a simple explanation of how this branch of medicine works so that it may be safely used for self-care and first aid in simple situations. Homoeopathy is as complex a study as any branch of medicine but its rudiments can be presented to the layman in a non-technical way, and that is what this Handbook seeks to do.

The Handbook's second purpose is to supply basic information about the practice of Homoeopathy in Britain today. It lists hospitals, organisations, publications etc, as sources from which further assistance and information may be sought.

Homoeopathy is practised by qualified doctors worldwide and has become recognised over the years as an effective and inherently safe form of medical treatment. The fact that homoeopathic remedies are without side effects and are safe, even for small children, makes them eminently suitable for self-medication in the treatment of common afflictions. Of particular help in this regard are the sections in the handbook headed 'Symptoms Guide to the Selection of a Medicine' and 'How to Use Homoeopathic Medicines'. Their purpose is to make the process of self-treatment as simple and as straightforward as possible.

Although the homeopathic doctor and pharmacist have at their disposal many more remedies than those listed, the selection in the Handbook provides the basis for a family medicine chest capable of dealing effectively with the common ailments and conditions to which nearly all of us are prone from time to time. From the practical point of view, the list has also been restricted to those remedies that are widely obtainable from pharmacies and health stores.

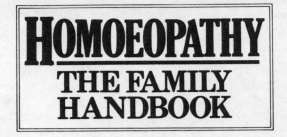

HOMOEOPATHY
THE FAMILY HANDBOOK

What is Homoeopathy?

The basic principle of Homoeopathy has been known since the time of the ancient Greeks. Derived from the Greek word 'Homoios' meaning 'like', Homoeopathy is the medical practice of treating like with like *similia similibus curentur*. That is to say, treating disease with substances that produce in a healthy person symptoms similar to those displayed by the person who is ill.

Current medical opinion believes that symptoms are caused by the disease; in contrast, Homoeopathy sees the symptoms as a positive sign of the body reacting against the disease as it attempts to overcome it and seeks to stimulate rather than suppress this reaction.

HOW HOMOEOPATHY BEGAN

In the eighteenth-century, Dr Samuel Hahnemann, convinced that existing medical practices did more harm than good, began to look for an alternative which would be safe, gentle and effective. Appalled by the medical procedures of the day, he believed that human beings have an innate capacity for healing themselves. He reasoned that instead of suppressing symptoms he should seek to stimulate them and so encourage and assist the body's natural healing process.

Basing his work on the 'like cures like' principle, Hahnemann found he could produce effective remedies by greatly diluting substances which in large doses would have created symptoms similar to those seen in the patient. Hahnemann had already discovered that a small dose of cinchona (quinine) in a healthy person produced the symptoms of malaria. A number of systematic experiments followed this discovery.

Hahnemann found that remedies obtained from animal, vegetable, mineral and more rarely biological materials were very effective in extreme dilutions. This was especially apparent in the case of poisons which often produced symptoms similar to those of certain illnesses and which, in very diluted doses, suggested themselves as remedies on the 'like cures like' principle.

Over a long period Hahnemann and his followers took small doses of various substances, carefully noting the symptoms they produced. These were called 'provings'. Subsequently, patients suffering from similar symptoms were treated with these substances. The results were usually encouraging and often remarkable.

Hahnemann then worked to establish the smallest effective dose as he realised this was the best way to avoid side effects. In so doing he unexpectedly discovered that the more a remedy was diluted, the more effective it became. Thus, by trial and by perseverance, Hahnemann had finally arrived at his goal – an alternative form of medical treatment that was both effective and safe.

PRINCIPLES OF HOMOEOPATHY

Homoeopathy is essentially a natural healing process in which the remedies assist the patient to regain health by stimulating the body's natural healing forces. The remedies appear to trigger this healing response in the body, leading to a correction of the illness.

Homoeopathy also concentrates on treating the patient rather than the disease, one of its principles is that a person's response to a disease varies according to his or her basic temperament. It follows, therefore, that a homoeopathic doctor will not automatically prescribe a specific remedy for a specific illness. Instead he will try to build up a picture of the patient's temperament and responses to certain conditions, so that he can prescribe for that individual. Because it is the patient who is being treated and not the disease, patients with the same ailment may often require different remedies. On the other hand, another group of patients experiencing different ailments could well benefit from the same remedy.

To summarise, by close observation and careful experiment Hahnemann established the three principles of Homoeopathy:

1 A medicine which in large doses produces the symptoms of a disease will in small doses cure that disease.

2 By extreme dilution, the medicine's curative properties are enhanced and all the poisonous or undesirable side effects are lost.

3 Homoeopathic medicines are prescribed individually by the study of the whole person, according to his or her basic temperament and response.

HOMOEOPATHY PROMOTES NATURAL HEALING

Homoeopathy is essentially natural healing. The remedy assists the patient to regain health by stimulating nature's vital forces of recovery. Plenty of rest and appropriate diet in satisfactory surroundings help recovery. In certain cases, especially in chronic illness, sufferers must be patient and give Homoeopathy time to take effect. Rapid results are often achieved in cases of acute illness but where a patient's vitality is low the treatment may be long term. If, as sometimes happens, irreversible body changes are present, other forms of medical or surgical treatment may be necessary. Once these have been given, homoeopathic medicines will help to prevent deterioration or recurrence.

Homoeopathic physicians do not underrate the value of surgery in advanced cases. They do, however, suggest that if homoeopathic treatment were started earlier far fewer cases would need the skill of the surgeon. Some of the happiest results of homoeopathic treatment can be seen in babies and children, where natural vitality is at its highest. Infrequent high potencies of a well-chosen remedy can set a child's feet firmly on the way to health. The effective treatment of children and animals gives conclusive proof that homoeopathic cures are not, as it is sometimes suggested, purely psychological.

Homoeopathy is not a cure-all, nor is it an elixir of life. Rather it is an idea, a way of looking at people in their surroundings and helping them to increase their sense of harmony and well-being. Homoeopathy does not reject the great discoveries of modern science, only their commercial abuse, and in many cases it is complementary to the newer methods of modern medical practice. In its present form Homoeopathy has stood the test of time. Today it has been highly developed in many countries to the extent that it is formally accepted as a safe and effective form of medical treatment that stands in its own right.

In Britain homoeopathy has been favoured by various members of the Royal Family; it is recognised by Act of Parliament and homoeopathic medicines are available on prescription under the National Health Service.

Questions and Answers

1 IS HOMOEOPATHY SAFE?
Homoeopathic medicines are not harmful because they are so greatly diluted. They are safe, non-toxic, and non-addictive. They are prepared in Medicines Control Agency licensed laboratories to stringent standards of quality.

2 IS HOMOEOPATHY EFFECTIVE?
Since the success of homoeopathic treatment of cholera and typhoid was demonstrated in the early nineteenth century, homoeopathy has proved effective for millions of people world-wide. It has often succeeded where other forms of treatment have failed.

3 IS HOMOEOPATHY OFFICIALLY RECOGNISED?
Homoeopathy was recognised by Act of Parliament in 1948, and accepted as a safe alternative form of medical treatment. It is practised by doctors who are fully qualified through conventional medical training and recognised by the General Medical Council. Homoeopathic prescriptions are available under the National Health Service.

4 WHERE CAN ONE RECEIVE HOMOEOPATHIC TREATMENT?
There are five homoeopathic hospitals in the National Health Service – London, Glasgow, Liverpool, Bristol and Tunbridge Wells and there are also some homoeopathic clinics. An increasing number of doctors practise Homoeopathy in Great Britain today; addresses can be obtained from organisations such as the British Homoeopathic Assocation.

5 HOW LONG SHOULD A HOMOEOPATHIC CONSULTATION LAST?
The first consultation, which is the longest, should on average last anything from three-quarters of an hour to an hour. This

is because the homoeopathic doctor needs to form a detailed picture of the patient; the patient's colouring, reaction to food and drink, hot and cold weather etc; and a full medical history are all recorded and taken into account. Then, when the doctor comes to prescribe a homoeopathic medicine he or she will choose one which matches the patient and the ailment. Subsequent consultations are usually much shorter.

6 WITH WHICH DISEASES CAN HOMOEOPATHY DEAL?

Homoeopathic medicine is a complete and scientific form of medicine. It appears to work by triggering a healing response in the body which leads to a correction of the disease. Therefore, as the patient regains health, the symptoms disappear. This can happen whatever the disease, although ideally the procedure needs the expert guidance of a qualified homoeopathic doctor. If the disease is incurable, the same medicine which fits the patient may ease considerably the symptoms, even if it does not lead to a cure.

7 WHERE SHOULD ONE STORE HOMOEOPATHIC MEDICINES?

Homoeopathic medicines should be stored in a cool place, away from strong sunlight. They should also be kept away from strong smelling substances, such as peppermint, perfume and especially camphor. **Do not** transfer medicines to a container that has held another homoeopathic medicine.

8 HOW LONG CAN THE MEDICINES BE STORED?

Properly stored homoeopathic medicines have an indefinite shelf life. However, it is better to change a medicine after five years.

9 HOW DOES ONE TAKE THE MEDICINES?

Homoeopathic medicines are available in different forms such as powders, granules, liquids, suppositories and tablets. Tablets are the most common form of medicine available. **They should not be handled.** Tip the tablets into a clean teaspoon and then drop them into the mouth to be chewed or sucked. Do not take them with food or drink.

10   HOW OFTEN SHOULD ONE TAKE THE TABLETS?
In acute conditions, two tablets should be taken every two hours for up to six times a day. Thereafter, two tablets taken three times daily until better. In chronic conditions, two tablets are taken three times daily for one week. Repeat in ten days if required. (For children and infants, the dose is one tablet crushed).

11   WHEN SHOULD ONE STOP TAKING THE TABLETS?
If an improvement in the symptoms is noted, then increase the interval between doses. If the improvement continues, stop dosing completely. If the symptoms return, restart the treatment.

12   FOR HOW LONG SHOULD ONE TRY A MEDICINE BEFORE SEEING A RESULT?
Whatever the symptoms, some feeling of improvement should be felt within one week, even though the symptoms may remain. If there is no improvement two weeks after starting the treatment another medicine should be considered.

13   CAN ONE TAKE HOMOEOPATHIC MEDICINE WITH ORDINARY DRUGS?
It is safe to do so, although any side-effects caused by the ordinary drug may complicate the symptom picture and make the correct choice of a homoeopathic medicine more difficult. **ALWAYS** follow your doctor's advice.

14   CAN MORE THAN ONE HOMOEOPATHIC MEDICINE BE TAKEN AT A TIME?
It is best to avoid this. Taking more than one medicine at a time makes it difficult to assess results.

15   IF THE SYMPTOMS BECOME WORSE WHEN FIRST TAKING A HOMOEOPATHIC MEDICINE IS IT ALL RIGHT OR DOES THIS INDICATE THE WRONG CHOICE OF MEDICINE?
Homoeopathic medicines seek to stimulate symptoms, not suppress them so that the body will overcome the disease

naturally. Therefore, if symptoms are 'aggravated' briefly, this usually means the medicine is working.

16   DO STRONG FLAVOURS, OR FOOD IN GENERAL, AFFECT THE ACTION OF THE MEDICINES?

It is best to take the medicines between meals, leaving at least one hour before or after taking food. It is also advisable to avoid strongly flavoured food or beverages, coffee for example. The use of flavoured toothpastes should also be avoided.

17   IS IT SAFE TO TAKE HOMOEOPATHIC MEDICINES DURING PREGNANCY?

The safety of homoeopathic medicines is well known. However, the law prohibits any medicine manufacturer from claiming that a medicine is safe during pregnancy. For guidance consult a qualified homoeopathic doctor.

18   ARE HOMOEOPATHIC MEDICINES SAFE IN THE TREATMENT OF CHILDREN?

Yes. They can be given safely, even to the youngest infant.

19   WHAT POTENCY SHOULD ONE USE?

The question of potency causes more confusion than any other. The most important thing to remember is that it is the selection of the right remedy that is of the greatest importance. The 6th potency is the most easily available and can be used in a large majority of cases. If the correct remedy is chosen, the results will be good.

20   IS A 'HIGH' POTENCY STRONGER THAN A LOW POTENCY?

Homoeopathy is a QUALITATIVE treatment and the normal meaning of 'strength' is inappropriate. Use the 6th potency for common ailments and leave the complications of potency to the physicians.

21   WHY IS IT NO LONGER POSSIBLE TO OBTAIN SOME LOW POTENCIES OF CERTAIN SUBSTANCES?

The introduction of Prescription Only Medicine (POM) Regulations means that a large number of substances at potencies below 6x can now be supplied ONLY on receipt of a valid prescription. Anyone wishing more detailed information on these regulations may obtain a copy from Her Majesty's Stationery Office.

22 SOME MEDICINES NOW CARRY A WARNING TO CONSULT A DOCTOR BEFORE TAKING THE MEDICINES. ARE THESE MEDICINES UNSAFE?
No, the medicines are safe; the warning is a legal requirement for all medicines. Homoeopathy has no exemption from the regulations designed to control the use of allopathic medicines.

23 HOMOEOPATHY IS SAID TO TREAT PATIENTS, NOT DISEASES. WHY THEN ARE THERE HOMOEOPATHIC MEDICINES FOR INDIGESTION, COLDS, 'FLU ETC?
There are various homoeopathic substances which have a very specific application in certain situations and so will treat, successfully, a large cross-section of the population. Many people have been introduced to the larger area of comprehensive homoeopathy by the successful results they have obtained from the use of these 'speciality' medicines.

24 ARE THE BACH REMEDIES HOMOEOPATHIC?
The preparation of the Bach remedies differs fundamentally from that of homoeopathic *potentisation*. Dr Bach at one time did research at The Royal London Homoeopathic Hospital which may be why this question is often asked. The use and prescription of these remedies is based upon mental symptoms (grief, anxiety, stress etc), whereas Homoeopathy takes both the physical and mental aspects of the patient into account.

25 ARE HOMOEOPATHY AND HERBAL MEDICINE RELATED?
There are homoeopathic remedies which are herbal in origin: Arnica for example, but they are not used or prepared in the same way as herbal medicines.

26 ARE ANIMALS USED IN HOMOEOPATHIC RESEARCH?

No. Homoeopathic remedies are developed using a process known as 'proving'. Here the symptoms the remedies produce in healthy people are noted so that, according to the basic principle of Homoeopathy, the same substances may be used to treat the same symptoms in a sick person. Animal tests are therefore not necessary, or even relevant.

27 CAN ANIMALS BE TREATED BY HOMOEOPATHY?

Homoeopathy is as effective for animals as it is for humans. There is an increasing number of veterinary surgeons practising Homoeopathy in the United Kingdom. Addresses are available from the British Homoeopathic Association.

28 HOW DO I KNOW IF A HOMOEOPATH IS PROPERLY QUALIFIED?

Doctors who have qualified in homoeopathy at either the Faculty of Homoeopathy in London or in Glasgow will have the initials MFHom or FFHom (Member/Fellow of the Faculty of Homoeopathy) after their names. For professional homoeo-paths who are not doctors, check that they are RSHom (registered with the Society of Homoeopaths).

How to Select and Use Homoeopathic Medicines

This guide to Self-Treatment relates to ailments which are usually treated at home. However, it cannot be over-emphasised that with chronic conditions or where the symptoms are serious or prolonged a qualified doctor should be seen.

1 Note your main symptoms and any strong likes and dislikes that may arise from them.
2 Study the SYMPTOMS GUIDE to find a selection of medicines from which you can make your choice.
3 Study the MEDICINE PICTURES carefully and select the medicine which most closely matches your symptoms.
4 You do not have to experience ALL the symptoms listed under a medicine nor need you exhibit all the likes or dislikes mentioned; they are often expressed as an extreme which may not always apply. Simply try to match up with the set of symptoms most similar to yours.
5 When treating simple, everyday ailments it is recommended that the 6th potency is used. This is the potency which is most easily available from your local pharmacy or health food store.
6 **Dosage:** The suggested dosage is two tablets for adults, one tablet for a child and one tablet, finely crushed, for an infant.
Frequency: In acute conditions every two hours for six doses, then three times a day, between meals until relief is obtained. Watch the response to each dose.
When improvement is evident, increase the interval between doses. Continue for two more days then STOP. Repeat only if the original symptoms recur.

8 If symptoms are somewhat increased do not be alarmed; this indicates that the medicine is working. Postpone the next dose until this increase or 'aggravation', as it is known, has passed.

9 Keep the medicines in a cool, dark place and away from strong smelling substances (camphor etc).

10 **To obtain the best absorption, tablets should be sucked or chewed, not swallowed whole.** They should also be taken apart from food or drink and dissolved on a clean tongue when the mouth is free from the effects of tobacco or strongly flavoured toothpastes.

11 **Always avoid handling the tablets;** they should be tipped into a clean teaspoon and then dropped into the mouth.

12 Always replace the cap of one container before opening another; this is to avoid cross-contamination of the medicines.

As with every new skill, practice and familiarity improves the performance. The better you get to know the medicines and your own reactions, the more accurate will be your selection and the more effective you will find the medicines.

IMPORTANT: **If symptoms are serious, prolonged or unusual, you should contact a qualified doctor.**

List of Medicines in Common Use

The following medicines are the most commonly used and most easily obtainable. Some medicines that are frequently recommended are not included in this list as generally they can be obtained only from specialist homoeopathic pharmacies.

Aconitum napellus
(**Aconite**)

Actaea racemosa
(**Actaea rac**)

Apis mellifica
(**Apis mel**)

Argentum Nitricum
(**Argent Nit**)

Arnica montana
(**Arnica**)

Arsenicum Album
(**Arsen Alb**)

Belladonna
(**Belladonna**)

Bryonia Alba
(**Bryonia**)

Calcarea Carbonica
(**Calc Carb**)

Calcarea Fluorica
(**Calc Fluor**)

Calcarea Phosphorica
(**Calc Phos**)

Cantharis vesicatoria
(**Cantharis**)

Carbo vegetabilis
(**Carbo veg**)

Cuprum Metallicum
(**Cuprum Met**)

Drosera rotundifolia
(**Drosera**)

Euphrasia officinalis
(**Euphrasia**)

Ferrum Phosphoricum
(**Ferrum Phos**)

Gelsemium sempervirens
(**Gelsemium**)

Graphites
(**Graphites**)

Hamamelis virginica
(**Hamamelis**)

Hepar Sulphuris
(**Hepar Sulph**)

Hypericum perforatum
(**Hypericum**)

Ignatia amara
(**Ignatia**)

Ipecacuanha
(**Ipecac**)

Kalium Bichromicum
(**Kali Bich**)

Kalium Phosphoricum
(**Kali Phos**)

Lycopodium clavatum
(**Lycopodium**)

Mercurius Solubilis
(**Merc Sol**)

Natrum Muriaticum
(**Natrum Mur**)

Nux vomica
(**Nux vom**)

Phosphorus
(**Phosphorus**)

Pulsatilla nigricans
(**Pulsatilla**)

Rhus toxicodendron
(**Rhus tox**)

Ruta graveolens
(**Ruta grav**)

Sepia
(**Sepia**)

Silicea
(**Silica**)

Sulphur
(**Sulphur**)

Thuja occidentalis
(**Thuja**)

The following remedies are also included which can be obtained from a homoeopathic pharmacy:

Ledum
Calendula Tincture
Causticum
Chamomilla
Urtica Urens Tincture

Symptoms Guide to the Selection of a Medicine

To select an appropriate medicine, consult the Symptons Guide and then refer to the list of medicines to find the one which most closely relates to the symptoms and to any likes or dislikes that arise.

Medicines for each ailment are listed alphabetically and not in order of suitability. In many cases there are other homoeopathic preparations which would be effective. However, those suggested have been selected as being most widely available.

It cannot be over-emphasised that this guide to self-treatment relates to ailments which are usually treated at home. **If symptoms are serious or prolonged, consult a qualified doctor.**

ABDOMINAL PAIN
Any abdominal pain lasting several hours, or of sudden onset accompanied by vomiting. Go to bed. If thirsty take small sips of water. Apply a covered hot water bottle to the painful area. If the pain persists, treat for shock and **get medical aid**.

TREATMENT	*Lycopodium, Nux vom*
Lycopodium	Bloated feeling after a light meal or after eating too much with excessive rumbling and flatulence.
Nux vom	Flatulence and swelling of the abdomen with colic pains, usually after over-eating and too much alcohol.

ABSCESS
An inflamed spot, swelling or boil containing pus. Apply a covered hot water bottle to the area or a compress of gauze saturated with a solution of *Hypericum Tincture* or *Calendula*

Tincture using two drops to one tablespoonful of water. If the abscess or boil is spreading, get medical aid.

TREATMENT	*Hepar Sulph, Silica*
Hepar Sulph	Where the abscess is burning, throbbing and extremely sensitive to touch.
Silica	When the discharge is slow to clear. The painful abscess feels cold. (Hepar Sulph feels hot)

BEDWETTING *See* URINE (INCONTINENCE OF)

BILIOUSNESS
Nausea, abdominal discomfort, headache and constipation.

TREATMENT	*Bryonia, Nux vom*
Bryonia	Vomiting of bile and water immediately after eating. Food lies heavily in the stomach.
Nux vom	Sour taste and nausea in the morning, after over-eating and from too much alcohol.

BITES AND STINGS *See* FIRST AID SECTION

BLACK EYE *See* FIRST AID SECTION

BLISTERS *See* FIRST AID SECTION

BOILS
This is an acute suppurative swelling under the skin, usually round and hard, and may discharge pus. Do not squeeze a boil.

TREATMENT	*Belladonna, Hepar Sulph, Silica*
Belladonna	Painful, dry and burning hot, with a red, shining, inflamed base. Pus forms rapidly.

Hepar Sulph	To mature the boil which is intolerably painful to touch and hot.
Silica	Small wounds which are difficult to heal and suppurate profusely. The boil is cold. (*Hepar Sulph* is hot).

BRAIN FAG *See* EXHAUSTION – MENTAL

BRONCHITIS

Acute bronchitis is an inflammation of the large air tubes in the chest and usually follows influenza and colds. It is marked by aching and tightness of the chest, shortness of breath and chest pain on coughing. **If there is chest pain or shortness of breath on movement or exertion, do not delay in getting medical aid.**

TREATMENT	*Aconite, Bryonia, Ipecac, Phosphorus*
Aconite	For early stages, with feverish nervous restlessness. Awakening in first sleep with short dry cough, causing severe pain and much tossing about.
Bryonia	Acute bronchitis, with dry hacking cough as if coming from the stomach. Entering a warm room from the cold excites a cough.
Ipecac	Spasmodic cough comes on quickly with rattling of mucus in the chest. There is an inclination to vomit but without nausea.
Phosphorus	Hoarseness and loss of voice, cannot speak above a whisper. Cough dry, tickling and with tightness across the chest.

BRUISES *See* FIRST AID SECTION

BURNS *See* FIRST AID SECTION

CARBUNCLE
Inflammation of a localised area of tissue, usually consisting of a cluster of suppurating boils

TREATMENT	*Arsen Alb, Hepar Sulph, Silica*
Arsen Alb	Large painful, inflamed carbuncle, with burning piercing pain even during sleep.
Hepar Sulph	To promote the discharge of pus. The carbuncle is extremely painful to touch and cannot bear the contact of the dressing.
Silica	Intensely painful, tending to recur, slow to heal and discharging a foul smelling greenish pus.

CATARRH
Inflammation of the mucous membrane which lines the air passages of the head, nose and throat.

TREATMENT	*Arsen Alb, Kali Bich, Pulsatilla*
Arsen Alb	Copious, clear and burning watery discharge. Sneezing, with watery eyes. Feels chilly, craves heat.
Kali Bich	Thick, greenish-yellow, tough, stringy and ropy discharge. Mucus difficult to detach.
Pulsatilla	Catarrh is variable, may be clear, thick and profuse, with greenish or yellow mucus. Suitable for chronic catarrhs.

CHICKEN POX
An infectious disease spread by contact. Starts with a crop of red spots which blister and form scabs which drop off after about ten days. Rash appears ten to twenty-one days after contact. It covers most of the head and body. Finger nails should be cut to avoid damage from scratching. **Get medical aid.**

TREATMENT	*Belladonna, Rhus tox*

Belladonna	Restlessness with burning hot skin. Face flushed and covered with deep red spots.
Rhus tox	Face and body covered with a red rash. There is intense itching and burning, with no relief from scratching. An ideal remedy at the beginning of the rash.

COLD SORES *See* HERPES SIMPLEX

COLLAPSE *See* FIRST AID SECTION

COMMON COLD AND INFLUENZA

Inflammation of the nose and throat with headache, fever, and aching muscles. Drink plenty of fluids and have at least one day in bed.

TREATMENT	*Aconite, Gelsemium, Natrum Mur*
Aconite	In the early stages of a cold of sudden onset and after exposure to cold wind. Sneezing and burning of the throat and mouth. Thirsty for cold drinks.
Gelsemium	Influenza, colds, chills play up and down the spine. Face hot and flushed, throat dry, burning and tight, but not thirst.
Natrum Mur	Frequent colds, with violent sneezing and copious flow of tears. Inflamed nose with profuse discharge of clear watery mucus.

CONJUNCTIVITIS

Inflammation of the delicate membrane covering the eye, and lining the eye lids.

TREATMENT	*Euphrasia*
Euphrasia	Inflammation of the eye and eyelids with continuous flow of burning tears and extreme sensitivity to light.

To prepare an eye lotion – Add two drops of *Euphrasia Tincture* to two tablespoons of water – **previously boiled and cooled**. Bathe the eyes daily with this lotion using a sterile eyebath. If the use of an eyebath is not convenient, use an eye dropper and pour over the eye.

COUGHS
See also BRONCHITIS

TREATMENT	*Aconite, Bryonia, Drosera*
Aconite	Constant hard, dry croupy cough, causes distress. Awakening in first sleep with short dry cough, patient sits up for relief.
Bryonia	Dry painful, shaking cough as if coming from the stomach.
Drosera	Sudden throat tickle and violent spasms of coughing, retching, gagging and vomiting. The spasms follow each other so rapidly that breathing can be difficult.

CRAMP
Most cramps come on for no apparent reason and often occur in bed. Cramp may occur after chilling, as in swimming, or from loss of body salt after vomiting, sweating or diarrhoea.

TREATMENT	*Cuprum Met*
Cuprum Met	Spasmodic cramp in the calves, the feet and toes, also the fingers, groin and abdomen.

CUTS AND WOUNDS *See* FIRST AID SECTION

CYSTITIS
Inflammation of the urinary bladder.

TREATMENT	*Belladonna, Cantharis, Lycopodium, Pulsatilla*
Belladonna	Uncontrollable dribbling of burning urine while standing or walking. Pains come and go suddenly. After passing urine, strains to pass more.
Cantharis	Violent straining to urinate, with painful discharge of urine drop by drop; doubles up with pain. The urge to urinate is worse when standing or walking, but eased when sitting.
Lycopodium	Urge to urinate, must wait a long time before it will pass. Urine cloudy with a red sand-like sediment.
Pulsatilla	Great urgency to urinate, impossible to delay. When going to urinate there is a feeling as if it will gush away. There is dribbling of urine on slightest provocation, such as coughing, sneezing or laughing

DIARRHOEA

Repeated loose, soft or liquid stools, may be caused by excitement, over-eating or infection.

TREATMENT	*Argent Nit, Arsen Alb*
Argent Nit	Diarrhoea immediately after eating sweets or drinking. Stools are greenish (like chopped spinach), with a foul shreddy mucus. Diarrhoea, retching and vomiting are brought on by emotional excitement and anticipation of future events.
Arsen Alb	Burning watery dark green stools with a foul greenish slimy mucus. Diarrhoea from fruit and vegetables and associated with tainted food and alcohol abuse.

DIZZINESS

Also known as GIDDINESS

TREATMENT	*Aconite, Argent Nit, Gelsemium*
Aconite	Especially on rising after lying down. May come on suddenly after a fright or shock accompanied by nausea and a staggering to the right.
Argent Nit	When looking up or down from a height or when over water. Usually accompanied by trembling and noises in the ears.
Gelsemium	Starts at the back of the head and causes a feeling of unsteadiness as if about to fall. Is increased by sudden movement of the head and may be accompanied by blurred vision.

EARACHE

If there is something in the ear, **get medical aid.**

TREATMENT	*Belladonna, Hepar Sulph*
Belladonna	Throbbing after standing in cold with head uncovered. Stinging in and behind the ear, with flushed redness, a great heat and intense throbbing.
Hepar Sulph	Sharp pain with great tenderness to touch, and discharge of offensive pus.

ECZEMA

Inflammation of the skin, usually red, itchy and painful, with tiny blisters oozing fluid and later crusting.

TREATMENT	*Graphites, Rhus tox, Sulphur*
Graphites	Itchy moist eczema, oozing a sticky honey-like discharge which may occur on any part of the body but especially the face, head and behind the ears. A scabby eruption may appear, the scab of which can be easily torn off leaving a raw bleeding surface.
Rhus tox	Itching over the whole body, especially where there is hair. Dry red itchy eczema of the hands and wrists forming small blisters.

Sulphur	Profuse itching, burning and tingling. An uncontrollable desire to scratch causes painful burning soreness. The skin is rough, red and painful.

EXHAUSTION – MENTAL

Characterised by undue tiredness on slight exertion. Loss of appetite and sleep, an inability to concentrate and feeling of being ill

TREATMENT	*Argent Nit, Gelsemium, Kali Phos*
Argent Nit	General trembling weakness and nervous restlessness, with sighing and palpitation. Always in a hurry and accomplishing nothing.
Gelsemium	Mentally dull and sluggish. Drowsiness and relaxed weak muscles. Desire to be left alone and to be quiet. Fear of crowds. Excitement in anticipation of news causes diarrhoea.
Kali Phos	After moderate mental effort. Nervous exhaustion, dread, night terrors, depressed and irritable.

EXHAUSTION – PHYSICAL

TREATMENT	*Arnica, Arsen Alb*
Arnica	For conditions induced by excessive physical effort. The body feels tired and aches as if it has been beaten, the limbs feel bruised when resting or moving. This may cause lassitude to the point of scarcely being able to stand. There may be sleeplessness from being too tired.

A hot bath will help to soothe your aching joints; add two teaspoonfuls of Arnica Tincture to the bath; in the case of tired and aching feet, add one teaspoon of Arnica Tincture to a foot-bath of hot water.

Arsen Alb   After effects of sickness, diarrhoea and vomiting. Great weakness and nervous prostration. There may be much chilliness and sweating with great thirst and dryness of the skin.

FEAR
Any persistent abnormal dread or aversion. Apprehension of pain. After any emotional upset or period of anger. See also **FRIGHT** (FIRST AID SECTION)

TREATMENT   *Aconite, Argent Nit, Arsen Alb*
Aconite   Fear of crowds, fear of space, fear of dark. Frantic impatience with great intolerance.
Argent Nit   Fear of failure, especially examinations (also *Gelsemium*). Fear of being forsaken. Fear upon setting out on a journey. Fear of being in an enclosed space.
Arsen Alb   Fear of being alone, fear of the dark, and of ghosts. Fear of guilt, patient feels he has upset or offended someone.

FOOD POISONING
Acute infection of the intestines usually caused by infected or decayed food, faulty kitchen hygiene, or by not covering or refrigerating food during hot weather.

TREATMENT   *Arsen Alb*
Arsen Alb   Violent diarrhoea and frequent stools, with nausea and vomiting. Caused by eating tainted meat, fruit, fish and vegetables.

FRACTURES *See* FIRST AID SECTION

FRIGHT *See* FIRST AID SECTION

GIDDINESS *See* DIZZINESS

GOUT
Caused by an excess of uric acid in the tissues of the affected joint.

TREATMENT	*Arnica, Rhus tox, Urtica Urens (Tincture)*
Arnica	For chronic gout, with hot painful joints which are very tender and extremely sensitive if touched. Acts especially on the big toe.
Rhus tox	Hard painful swelling of the big toe joints, often mistaken for a bunion and frequently called 'rheumatic gout'.
Urtica Urens (Tincture)	Much benefit can be obtained by taking three drops of *Urtica Urens Tincture* in one teaspoonful of water three times a day.

HAEMORRHOIDS *See* PILES

HAYFEVER
An acute congestion of the nasal membrane, with running eyes, sneezing and catarrh.

TREATMENT	*Arsen Alb, Euphrasia, Pulsatilla*
Arsen Alb	Eyes burning hot with a flow of hot burning tears. Sneezing with no relief.
Euphrasia	Profuse nasal discharge during the day, nose blocked at night. Sensation of having sand in the eyes with a copious flow of burning tears.
Pulsatilla	Inflammation of eyes and the eyelids. Profuse discharge of thick yellow mucus. Itching and burning of the eyes compels rubbing and scratching.

HEADACHE

There are many and varied causes, such as: infection of the ears or throat, before a cold or fever or from fright or fear, anxiety and worry.

TREATMENT	*Belladonna, Ignatia, Natrum Mur*
Belladonna	Burning, violent throbbing headache with extremely sensitive scalp, accentuated by stooping and relieved by bending the head backwards.
Ignatia	Congestive, throbbing headache following grief or anger. Pain may extend to the eyes or the root of the nose and is associated with fiery zigzags and with blurring of vision.
Natrum Mur	Migraine–type of headache with frontal pain, throbbing or beating like little hammers, accompanied by nausea and vomiting. Spots or zigzags in front of the eyes and sometimes loss of vision.

HEARTBURN

INDIGESTION A burning sensation behind the breastbone, usually due to a return flow of acid into the food pipe. Normally this responds to a glass of milk or to indigestion tablets. If the heartburn is accompanied by pain in the neck or arm, it may be something other than indigestion – **get medical aid**.

TREATMENT	*Carbo veg, Lycopodium, Nux vom*
Carbo veg	Nausea, *waterbrash* (wind accompanied by an acid fluid in the mouth) and burning in the stomach. Constant belching, with the passing of offensive wind. Usually caused by over-indulgence in food and drink.
Lycopodium	Severe heartburn, prolonged and intolerable, extending to the top of the food pipe. *Waterbrash* is common, with a burning pain between the shoulder blades.

Nux vom	Acidity after too much coffee, alcohol and from over-eating. There is nausea, vomiting and retching but with ravenous hunger.

HERPES SIMPLEX
Clusters of small blisters, developing on the lips, nose and the mouth. Usually the result of the common cold and frequently called cold sores.

TREATMENT	*Natrum Mur, Rhus tox*
Natrum Mur	On the bends of the elbows and the knees. Eruptions on the mouth and lips, cold sores with blister spots. Swelling of the lower lip.
Rhus tox	Eruptions of burning pimples, around the lips and chin. Corners of the lips are burning, sore and ulcerated.

INCONTINENCE *See* URINE (INCONTINENCE OF)

INDIGESTION *See* HEARTBURN

INSOMNIA *See* SLEEPLESSNESS

ITCHING

TREATMENT	*Apis mel, Arsen Alb, Sulphur*
Apis mel	A rash with intolerable itching and burning. Extremely sensitive to heat, even the scalp is abnormally sensitive.
Arsen Alb	Itching and burning of dry scaly skin, relieved by rubbing but the burning continues. Craving for cold drinks.
Sulphur	Itching and burning of the skin. Scratching gives some feeling of pleasure and temporary relief, but afterwards there is aching,

burning and numbness, sometimes leading to ulceration.

JOINTS
Painful, swollen, inflamed or arthritic.

TREATMENT	*Apis mel, Rhus tox, Ruta grav*
Apis mel	Painful swollen arthritic joints, with burning and stinging pain. Stiffness in the neck and shoulder blades. Knees and feet stiff and swollen.
Rhus tox	Swelling and stiffness of joints, from sprains, over-stretching or over-lifting. Ankles swollen after sitting too long when travelling.
Ruta grav	Painful wrists, knuckles, knees and ankles, with or without swelling, but always feeling bruised.

LARYNGITIS
Acute or chronic inflammation of the vocal chords. Usually accompanied by hoarseness and loss of voice.

TREATMENT	*Causticum, Drosera, Phosphorus*
Causticum	Burning pain in the throat and the vocal chords with rawness, soreness, hoarseness and loss of voice, with a dry hollow irritating cough.
Drosera	With a deep bass voice, and a feeling of suffocation when talking or coughing. Tickling, coughing spasms follow each other so violently that breathing can be difficult.
Phosphorus	With a rough husky voice, cannot speak above a whisper. Loss of voice, from prolonged talking. Cough hard and dry with soreness of the chest.

LIVERISH

TREATMENT	*Aconite, Nux vom. Sulphur*
Aconite	Sudden inclination to violent vomiting with gagging and retching, usually after eating something sweetish or containing fat. All kinds of food and liquids taste bitter except water.
Nux vom	Constant nausea, inclined to vomit, especially in the morning, during a meal, and after eating or drinking alcohol. Liver inflamed with pain in the right side and right shoulder. Sensitivity to touch.
Sulphur	Jaundiced appearance. Excessively ravenous appetite. A need to eat frequently which, if ignored causes headache accompanied by vomiting.

LONELINESS

Can be long term and may be accentuated by a bereavement or domestic crisis.

TREATMENT	*Lycopodium, Pulsatilla*
Lycopodium	Feels extremely self-conscious, shuns crowds. Feels insecure unless there is someone in the house, but quite content to be alone in the next room. Apprehensive before an ordeal but rises to the occasion when it arrives.
Pulsatilla	Feels lonely unless constantly surrounded by people to give reassurance. Desire for affection and consolation.

LUMBAGO

The common problem of low back pain or ache, often incapacitating and paralysing, following strain, over-lifting, poor posture and exposure to cold and damp.

TREATMENT	*Bryonia, Calc Fluor, Rhus tox*
Bryonia	Shooting pains in the lower back and from the buttocks to the ankles. Pains are severe and violent, patient cannot keep still yet on movement cries out with worse pain. Eased by lying on the painful area.
Calc Fluor	Chronic lumbago from the least strain. Severe backache after long journeys. Worse when beginning to move but improved with continual movement.
Rhus tox	Pain after over-lifting or over-stretching. Lameness and stiffness with pain on first moving, especially after resting or getting up in the morning. Great restlessness and uneasiness, constantly changing position.

MEASLES

An acute contagious infectious disease of children, usually under the age of six. First symptoms similar to a severe cold – eyes pink and painful in bright light, runny nose, throat red and inflamed, hard dry cough. Affects neck, face, trunk, arms and legs. Child infectious from one – three weeks. Protect eyes from bright light. **Get medical aid**.

TREATMENT	*Euphrasia, Belladonna, Pulsatilla*
Euphrasia	For early stages. Streaming eyes and nose. Eyes painful in bright light, temperature is moderate.
Belladonna	For small, flat or raised spots, bright red, hot and dry. Eyes pink with dilated pupils. Throat sore, hot, no thirst. The child may appear to be very hot, be careful; cold air, cold draughts and cold applications can upset.
Pulsatilla	Red spots, itching and burning. Profuse discharge of hot tears. Sore, dry throat, dry mouth but no thirst, worse from heat. Cough may be troublesome all day and cease at night or cough may be worse

when lying down and have to sit up to get more air.

MEASLES – GERMAN
A mild form of viral infection also known as Rubella. Symptoms are similar to measles but the rash is usually the first sign. Fever, itching and swollen glands. Treatment as for measles. Infectious from two days before the rash appears and remaining so for a further three to four days. Incubation period two-three weeks. **Get medical aid.**

MENOPAUSE
Change of life – the period of cessation of menstruation.

TREATMENT	*Pulsatilla, Sepia*
Pulsatilla	Where there are hot flushes with profuse musty-smelling sweat. Relief derived from cold drinks even if not thirsty.
Sepia	Sudden attacks of hot flushes, redness of the face, sweating and a bearing down sensation. Inclined to be anxious and intolerant.

MENSTRUATION *See* PERIODS

MENTAL STRAIN *See* EXHAUSTION – MENTAL

MIGRAINE
A severe one-sided headache. There can be loss of vision with sickness and dizziness. If you find you are starting an attack, lie down in a darkened room. Every bad headache is not a migraine.

TREATMENT   *Kali Bich, Natrum Mur, Silica*

Kali Bich	Periodic intense headache, may be felt in a particular point. The migraine is preceded by loss of vision, and is accompanied by nausea and vomiting.
Natrum Mur	The migraine is severe and frontal, or maybe affecting one side, and with nausea and vomiting. Periodic recurrence is common with spots of fiery zigzags in front of the eyes and temporary loss of vision.
Silica	Chronic violent sick headache, with nausea and vomiting. The pain rises from the back of the neck, moving over the head to the eyes. There are sparks and specks before the eyes and dimness of vision.

MORNING SICKNESS
Nausea and vomiting of early pregnancy.

TREATMENT	*Ipecac, Nux vom*
Ipecac	For nausea with copious saliva and persistent vomiting which does not relieve the nausea. Constant nausea, with a clean tongue.
Nux vom	For nausea and vomiting every morning with much retching and gagging. The vomiting is distressing and difficult, but does give some relief.

MUMPS
An acute infectious disease characterised by swelling of the glands in front of and below the ears. Incubation period is 18–21 days. **Get medical aid.**

TREATMENT	*Belladonna, Merc Sol, Pulsatilla*
Belladonna	Right-sided mumps with fever, glowing redness and swelling of the neck glands. Burning heat of the face and neck, with or without redness, and very sensitive to cold.

Merc Sol	Painful stinging inflammation and swelling of the glands, especially the area below the right ear and right jaw. Pain in the cheek bones, very painful when blowing the nose.
Pulsatilla	Sharp pain in the jaws, with swelling of the neck glands. Temperature is high but feels chilly. Condition becomes worse with warmth. There is no thirst. There may be constant chilliness, even in a warm room, and a desire for fresh air.

NAPPY RASH

A temporary eruption on the skin of infants, localised to the areas covered by a nappy. It is caused by the irritants in decomposed urine.

TREATMENT	*Calendula cream, Hypericum and Calendula ointment* Keep the affected parts dry and clean with frequent changes of nappy. Apply a *Calendula cream*. If the skin is very dry, apply *Hypericum and Calendula Ointment*.

NAUSEA

A feeling of discomfort in the region of the stomach, with retching, a tendency to vomit, and profuse salivation and sweating.

TREATMENT	*Arsen Alb, Ipecac, Nux vom*
Arsen Alb	Excessive, with an inclination to vomit, and an unquenchable thirst. Drinks often but only a little at a time.
Ipecac	Sudden onset with copious saliva and empty belching, especially after drinking anything cold.
Nux vom	Continual, with an inclination to vomit. Nausea after a meal, with a flow back of food and liquid into the mouth.

NECK – STIFFNESS

May be due to muscular rheumatism or caused by draughts, exposure to cold, chill or tension.

TREATMENT	*Aconite, Actaea rac*
Aconite	With severe tearing pain at the nape of the neck and between the shoulder blades, with stiffness in the back. Onset sudden, after exposure to dry cold winds or excessive summer heat.
Actaea rac	Stiffness and cramp in the neck muscles, especially on moving the head or hands. Pain in the left shoulder after exposure to cold air.

NERVOUSNESS

Apprehension, uneasiness, panic, impatience and emotional upset.

TREATMENT	*Aconite, Argent Nit, Gelsemium, Natrum Mur*
Aconite	Very restless, anxious and will not be consoled. Fear of crowds, darkness and space. Attacks are violent and sudden.
Argent Nit	Nervous restlessness, impulsive and irrational, always in a hurry. Nervous anticipation of a coming event.
Gelsemium	As in stage-fright or before an examination. Fear of embarrassment.
Natrum Mur	Extreme sensitivity, with great desire to be left alone. Suffers silent grief and when alone is inclined to weep.

NETTLERASH

Urticaria – extremely itchy, red, raised blotchy rash – it is not infectious.

TREATMENT	*Apis mel, Lycopodium, Natrum Mur, Sulphur*
Apis mel	Violent rash all over the body, with swelling and stinging pain. Skin burns and itches, especially at night. Cannot tolerate any form of heat and there is no thirst.
Lycopodium	With large red weals or nodules, burning and itching on becoming warm during the day or in the evening before lying down.
Natrum Mur	Stinging and itching rash all over the body, with large red burning and smarting blotches, especially after a period of violent exercise. Frequently there is great thirst for tea.
Sulphur	Bright red rash with itching and tingling all over the body, with an uncontrollable desire to scratch which produces intense burning and smarting, sometimes with bleeding.

NEURALGIA
A spasm of severe pain, along the course of one or more nerves. The causes and varieties of neuralgia are very varied.

TREATMENT	*Actaea rac, Belladonna, Gelsemium*
Actaea rac	Neuralgia of the eyes, with a sensation as if the eyeballs were being pierced by needles. Neuralgia of the cheekbone, the pain passes off at night and returns next morning.
Belladonna	Nervous right-sided facial neuralgia, with violent cutting pains, twitching muscles, hot and burning red flushed face.
Gelsemium	Pains at the nape of the neck, the pain extends over the head causing pain in the forehead and eyeballs. This may be accompanied by numbness, nausea and vomiting.

NOSE BLEED *See* FIRST AID SECTION

PAINS
Burning and shooting.

TREATMENT	*Actaea rac, Apis mel, Hypericum, Sulphur*
Actaea rac	Like an electric shock, affecting neck, shoulders and lower back, worse in cold damp weather.
Apis mel	Like hot needles; shifting from place to place with widespread swelling and worse from heat.
Hypericum	Shooting and darting from the part affected. Useful for injured nerves especially spinal injury, puncture wounds from sharp objects or splinters.
Sulphur	General and local burning with excessive burning of the feet, while in bed. Pains are periodic, may occur every week or every two weeks.

PAINFUL HIP JOINT
Usually arthritic.

TREATMENT	*Bryonia, Rhus tox*
Bryonia	Joints painful, swollen and stiff, make stitching and tearing pain on movement. Worse from heat and eased by cold applications.
Rhus tox	Stiffness and pain when resting. Pain worse on rising but better for sustained movement. Worse from cold and damp, relief from hot applications.

PAINFUL KNEE JOINT
Usually arthritic.

TREATMENT	*Bryonia, Pulsatilla, Rhus tox*
Bryonia	Knee joint stiff and swollen, worse from movement and heat, better when resting, and after cold applications.
Pulsatilla	Knees crack frequently. Pains are cutting, stitching, tearing, wandering and variable. Worse from heat, better walking in cool air. Usually chilly and with no thirst.
Rhus tox	Worse when resting and on rising, but better after sustained movement. Made worse by cold draughts and dampness; relieved by hot applications.

PERIODS
The monthly menstrual period may be painful and with cramp, early or delayed, scanty or profuse.

TREATMENT	*Aconite, Actaea rac, Belladonna, Natrum Mur, Pulsatilla*
Aconite	Suppressed or delayed, from exposure to extreme cold or from cold feet. From fear, fright and shock.
Actaea rac	Early, profuse, dark clotted and offensive. May be irregular, scanty and delayed. Painful bearing down sensation in the lower part of abdomen, and low back pain, from one hip joint to the other.
Belladonna	Before the period there is fatigue, painful colic and loss of appetite. Periods bright red, too early, profuse, hot and with a violent bearing down sensation.
Natrum Mur	Irregular, usually profuse. Before the period, irritable and morose; at onset frequently sad; during, abdominal cramp. Every morning there is a bearing down sensation, compelled to sit down.
Pulsatilla	Painful, late, scanty, delayed, very changeable, flow stops and starts. Pain and nausea before the period. Suitable for pale

anaemic girls at puberty, who fail to men-
struate even if all the signs are present.

PILES
HAEMORRHOIDS – Varicose veins of the rectum, or anus.
If there is excessive bleeding and pain, get medical aid – the
skin may be torn.

TREATMENT	*Hamamelis, Nux vom, Sulphur*
Hamamelis	Bleeding profusely, with burning and sore-ness and a great urge to stool. The back feels as if it would break and the anus is sore, raw and itching.
Nux vom	Blind piles with shooting burning pain. Some time after stool there is burning, smarting and itching in the anus, usually worse after stool and after a meal.
Sulphur	Blind piles with burning and sharp pain in the anus, relieved when lying down but recurring when walking and on standing. Itching, burning and stinging at night.

PRICKLY HEAT *See* NETTLERASH

PSORIASIS
A chronic, frequently hereditary, skin condition. Characterised by dry, red, scaly and flaky areas. Usually involves
the scalp, elbows, knees and legs.

TREATMENT	*Arsen Alb, Graphites, Sulphur*
Arsen Alb	Skin dry as parchment, rough, scaly and cold with bluish spots. Burning and itching of small red pimples, usually covered with scurf. In chronic cases, the skin is thickened, burning and itching.
Graphites	Obstinate dryness of the skin, with itching and burning. The skin is dry and cracked,

the fissures itch, bleed, are very painful and discharge a sticky fluid.

Sulphur   Skin burning and dry, with crawling itch all over the body. Scratching gives temporary relief but is followed by burning pain and soreness. Patient cannot tolerate heat and dislikes extreme cold.

QUINSY
Inflammation and suppuration of the Tonsils

TREATMENT   *Belladonna, Hepar Sulph, Silica*

Belladonna   Sensation of enlarged tonsils, with dryness and burning, the formation of reddish white spots and tearing pain on swallowing. Neck glands hot and swollen.

Hepar Sulph   Tonsils enlarged, with swollen glands and a tendency to suppurate. Shooting pains into the ear. Speech difficult, swallowing almost impossible.

Silica   Suppurating tonsils, slow to heal. Neck glands swollen, swallowing painful and difficult. Numbness of the soft palate may cause food to be ejected through the nose.

RHEUMATISM
Inflammation of the muscles and the joints, with acute pain and swelling.

TREATMENT   *Actaea rac, Arnica, Bryonia, Rhus tox, Ruta grav*

Actaea rac   Pain in the muscles and joints of the neck and the back with severe pain in the back down to the thighs. Pains are like electric shocks.

Arnica   Pain in the joints of the arms, hands and wrists, with acute pain in the ball of the thumb. Aching over all the limbs as if bruised and broken.

Bryonia	Swelling of the right shoulder, upper arm, elbow and the upper part of the hands and their joints. Cracking of the hip joints when walking. Movement affects all joints.
Rhus tox	Severe stiffness of the neck, shoulder blades, hands and fingers, with tearing pains in the lower back, increased on resting. Pains are worse on starting to move and better on continued gentle movement.
Ruta grav	Painful wrists, the back of the hands and knuckles. Painful knees and feet, with or without swelling. Sciatic pain, with urge to walk, but the bruised feeling in the thighs makes movement very difficult. Knees inclined to give way when rising.

RUPTURE

Hernia. Treatment of rupture in the adult is a surgical procedure and the treatment suggested here can only be supportive. It must NOT be regarded as curative or a substitute for surgery.

TREATMENT	*Belladonna, Lycopodium, Nux vom*
Belladonna	Abdomen painfully tender and swollen with heat and burning. Colic pains come on quickly and pass off quickly, relieved by bending forward and may be accompanied by vomiting. Most frequently the right side is affected but it can affect the left side.
Lycopodium	Sensation of pressure in the region of the groin, as if a hernia were about to protrude on the right side. There is a great deal of noisy wind in the lower abdomen and in the area of the lower ribs.
Nux vom	A feeling of weakness in the groin, with swelling of the glands, as if a hernia was constricted and about to protrude. There is much flatulence and abdominal distension after eating.

SCALDS *See* FIRST AID SECTION

SCARS
Marks remaining after the healing of a wound.

TREATMENT	*Calc Fluor, Graphites*
Calc Fluor	Skin rough, dry, liable to chap and fissure, expecially the palms of the hands. Scars become unhealthy and break down. Suitable for adhesions after operations.
Graphites	Skin hard, very dry, rough and liable to crack, especially during the winter. Old scars tend to burn and may ulcerate and discharge a thick sticky fluid.

SCIATICA
Inflammation and pain anywhere along the path of the Sciatic nerve.

TREATMENT	*Arsen Alb, Ignatia, Rhus tox*
Arsen Alb	Pain at the neck of the thigh, shooting down to the knee, then to the ankle. In elderly people the pains are intermittent and the knees stiff.
Ignatia	With sharp cutting pains in the lower back, extending to the thighs. The attacks are preceded by coldness and shivering, and during the spasms is forced to get out of bed and walk around to obtain relief.
Rhus tox	With shooting and tearing pain in the hip joint, extending to the knee. There is involuntary limping and the pain is located mostly in the right knee. Always worse in cold, damp conditions and at night when resting.

SEASICKNESS *See* FIRST AID SECTION

SHINGLES
Groups of small blisters along the pathway of a nerve, usually caused by the chicken pox virus, extremely painful, mostly seen in elderly persons.

TREATMENT *Apis mel, Arsen Alb, Rhus tox*

Apis mel Blisters large and swollen, sometimes running together, with extreme burning and stinging pain, and a tendency to ulcerate. Relieved by cold applications.

Arsen Alb Skin red, with blisters running together. There is violent burning, and a foul discharge from the blisters. Relieved by hot applications.

Rhus tox With red, highly inflamed skin, covered with clear white blisters, burning hot and itchy, feeling as if pierced with red hot needles. Affecting the mouth, scalp and trunk. Greatly distressed and painful, yet unable to be still.

SHOCK *See* FIRST AID SECTION

SICKNESS *See* MORNING SICKNESS, NAUSEA, SEASICKNESS (FIRST AID SECTION)

SINUSITIS
Inflammation of a sinus, especially the frontal sinus. *See also* CATARRH, COMMON COLD, HAYFEVER *and* INFLUENZA

TREATMENT *Hepar Sulph, Kali Bich, Natrum Mur, Pulsatilla, Silica*

Hepar Sulph Inflammation and swelling of the nose, extremely painful to touch, with discharge of thick, yellow, offensive mucus. Sneezing and runny nose after exposure to cold, dry winds.

Kali Bich	Inflammation of the whole nasal mucous membrane with a discharge of thick, sticky, ropy yellow mucus. Inflamed frontal sinus, with pain shooting from roof of the nose to the eye, and accompanied by a frontal headache over the eye.
Natrum Mur	Excessive sneezing with profuse watery discharge, alternating with stoppage of the nose to the eye, and accompanied by a frontal headache over the eye.
Pulsatilla	Catarrhal inflammation of the nose with profuse thick, yellow, mild discharge. The discharge may alternate from side to side or there may be blockage, with frontal headache. Usually occurs in the evening and in the morning.
Silica	Frequent bouts of sneezing, with dry stuffed-up itchy nose. May be accompanied by a severe headache, from the nape of the neck over the head to above the eye.

SKIN
Unhealthy skin, sore etc – *See* BOILS, ECZEMA, NETTLERASH *and* PSORIASIS

SLEEPLESSNESS
May be caused by depression, excitement, nervous anticipation, over activity, restlessness or tension.

TREATMENT	*Aconite, Arnica, Nux vom, Sulphur, Thuja*
Aconite	From sudden nervous upset, fear or fright with great restlessness, anxiety, tossing about and undoing the bedclothes. Suitable for infants and elderly persons.
Arnica	From injuries and bruises and from being too tired. Body painful all over and bed feels very hard.

Nux vom	Due to overwork, especially working late at night, and from lack of exercise. May also be caused by indigestion, wind and too much alcohol.
Sulphur	From over-excitement and from a great flow of ideas. Is awakened by the slightest noise and remains wide awake for some time.
Thuja	Persistent with pain in the parts on which the patient is lying and with a sensation of coldness of the body. Eyes wide open and desire to sleep disappears once lying down.

SPRAINS AND STRAINS *See* FIRST AID SECTION

STINGS AND BITES *See* BITES AND STINGS – FIRST AID SECTION

STYE
A stye is an inflammation and suppuration on the edge of the eyelid, starting in a hair follicle at the base of an eyelash.

TREATMENT	*Graphites, Phosphorus, Pulsatilla, Silica*
Graphites	Chronic styes, may appear on both eyes, and discharge a sticky pus. Styes frequently appear on the lower lids and the edges can be covered with crusty scabs.
Phosphorus	Suppurating, burning styes, with yellowish eyeball. Eyelids are sticky in the morning. Objects appear to have a green or red halo. Profuse flow of tears when facing a wind.
Pulsatilla	General tendency to styes, with copious discharge of non-irritating, greenish yellow mucus. Styes with inflammation of the whole eye. Eyelids swollen, itchy, burning and sticking together at night.

Silica	Recurring styes, itching, burning and smarting with dryness as if there is sand or a splinter in the eye. Ulceration of the eyelids, very sticky in the morning.

SUNBURN *See* FIRST AID SECTION

SUNSTROKE *See* FIRST AID SECTION

SUPPURATION

TREATMENT	*Graphites, Hepar Sulph, Merc Sol, Silica, Sulphur*
Graphites	Unhealthy looking skin, dry, rough and liable to crack. Wounds and scratches become septic. Itchy blotches affecting face, chin and behind the ears with a thick, or watery, sticky fluid
Hepar Sulph	Chapped skin, with deep cracks, especially the hands and feet. Every little injury suppurates discharging a foul smelling pus. Ulcers may be surrounded by small pimples. All wounds are very sensitive and extremely painful to touch.
Merc Sol	Skin dirty yellow, chafed and sore. Small inflammatory swellings containing pus. The discharge is burning, has a foul odour and sometimes forms a crust. Itching is always inflamed by the heat of the bed.
Silica	A tendency to boils, usually in crops at the nape of the neck. Abscesses form and discharge a foul greenish fluid. There is a sensation of coldness in boils, ulcers and abscesses. Frequent ulceration of the nails.
Sulphur	Every little injury suppurates. Usually red itchy and hot round the edges. The skin is

dry, rough and scaly. Crops of itchy boils. Widespread itching, scratching may at first be pleasant, but leads to burning and smarting.

SYNOVITIS

Inflammation of a synovial membrane, usually painful on motion, characterised by a fluctuating swelling. Affects ligaments and tendons, all joints particularly wrists, elbows, knees and ankles. *See also* JOINTS

TREATMENT	*Apis mel, Belladonna, Pulsatilla, Rhus tox, Ruta grav*
Apis mel	Acute synovitis in the early stage, with the joint painful, hot and swollen; especially the white puffy swelling of the knee joint. Relieved by cold applications.
Belladonna	The knee joint, with intense inflammation, burning and stinging pain. When walking the joint feels as if it could give way.
Pulsatilla	Redness and swelling of the joints. Hot swelling of the elbow after a blow or a bruise. Knees hot, inflamed and swollen with shooting pains. Tearing pains in the limbs, shift rapidly from place to place.
Rhus tox	Hot, painful swelling and stiffness of the joints from over-stretching and over-lifting. Hot swelling of the hands and fingers. Wrenching pain and swelling around the ankles when resting on the feet or after sitting too long.
Ruta grav	Inflammation of the larger joints, especially the elbow as from a strain, or bruised after a blow. Pain in the forearms and in the bones, joints of the wrists, knuckles and hands. Usually when resting and on movement there is bruised pain in the hip joint, the knees and the bones of the legs.

TEETHING
The process of development and cutting of teeth. May be associated with disturbed sleep, restlessness and inflammation of the gums.

TREATMENT	*Aconite, Apis mel, Belladonna, Chamomilla*
Aconite	Child gnaws its fist, frets and cries. May be sleepless, but can be alert, alarmed or excited. Restless tossing at night accompanied by wailing.
Apis mel	Sudden involuntary grinding of teeth. Child is fidgety and tearful. Shrill sudden piercing screams while awake or sleeping. Retention of urine in infants – if this persists **get medical aid.**
Belladonna	This child suffers sudden attacks which cease just as suddenly. The face is very hot and red and pupils are dilated. Starts and wakes just when falling asleep.
Chamomilla	Sweating due to the pain from teething. Uneasy and anxious at night, tossing and requiring to drink often. Demands attention and wants to be carried. Inclined to be peevish and irritable. One cheek is red and hot, the other pale and cold. There may be diarrhoea with slimy greenish stools smelling of rotten eggs.

TENDINITIS
Inflammation of tendons and of tendon-muscles attachments.
See JOINTS and SYNOVITIS

THROAT
SORE THROAT – An inflamed and uncomfortable condition that may vary from a tickling sensation to painful swallowing or loss of voice.

TREATMENT	*Aconite, Apis mel, Arsen Alb, Belladonna, Hepar Sulph, Kali Bich, Merc Sol*
Aconite	Sudden onset of acute inflammation of the throat with fever, dry heat, burning thirst, painful swallowing and hoarseness or a dry croupy cough.
Apis mel	Throat swollen, with inflammation, redness, burning with stinging pains which extend to the ears. Inability to swallow and no thirst.
Arsen Alb	Great dryness, with extreme heat and burning in the throat and mouth. Continual drinking but swallowing is extremely difficult.
Belladonna	Throat painful, raw, sore and burning, chiefly on the right side. Highly inflamed, bright red and shining with a sensation of a lump, which causes hawking and shooting pains when swallowing.
Hepar Sulph	Painful throat with difficulty in swallowing. Prickly, shooting sensation in the throat as if from pins, fish bone or splinters, chiefly when coughing or swallowing.
Kali Bich	Sharp shooting pain in the left side of the throat extends to the ears and is relieved by swallowing. Sensation of a plug at the back of the throat which is not relieved by swallowing. Dryness and burning of the throat in the morning with an accumulation of tough, sticky mucus.
Merc Sol	Painful dryness of the throat but the mouth is full of saliva. Burning rawness and constant dryness of the throat usually the right side with the pain extending to the ears and accompanied by a copious flow of thin, foul-smelling saliva.

THRUSH
Infection of the mucous membrane of the mouth of infants
(and sometimes adults). Characterised by the formation of
reddish white spots in the mouth, followed by a shallow ulcer.
May be accompanied by fever, gastro-intestinal irritation.

TREATMENT	*Arsen Alb, Merc Sol, Natrum Mur, Sulphur*
Arsen Alb	The mouth is inflamed. Tongue bright red with silver white coating and small raised blisters at the tip. Mouth dry and burning. Craves ice or cold water but this upsets the stomach and is vomited at once.
Merc Sol	Sore mouth in children with reddish patches on the tongue, has a craving for fat and during teething the stools look like lumps of chalk. Mouth slimy with blisters on the inside of the cheek. Breath offensive. Profuse saliva at night.
Natrum Mur	Lips swollen with greater swelling of the lower lip followed by a large blister. Crack in the middle of the lower lip. Numbness of one side of the nose, of the lip and of the tongue. The tongue has painful burning blisters, or may be clean and shiny with froth on the edges. Reddish white spots in the mouth and on the tongue. Unquenchable thirst.
Sulphur	Reddish white blisters in the mouth. Profuse saliva with a foul taste. Lips dry, rough and cracked. Tongue white with a red tip. Bad odour from mouth after eating.

TINNITUS AURIUM
Noises in the ears, perceived only by the person affected and
may be buzzing, ringing, hissing, whistling etc. This condition
is usually due to a process of slow degeneration of the
auditory nerves. In such cases the remedies may only tempo-
rarily relieve the condition. **Get medical aid**.

TREATMENT	*Aconite, Graphites, Lycopodium, Phosphorus, Sulphur*
Aconite	All types of noise intolerable. Music unbearable – induces sadness
Graphites	Buzzing and rumbling like thunder in the ears. Sensation as if the left ear were filled with water. Whistling and crackling in the ears when eating or moving the jaw.
Lycopodium	Roaring, humming and a sensation of hot blood rushing in the ears, particularly the right ear. Music causes fatigue. In the evening, hears music heard during the day.
Phosphorus	Frequent buzzing, roaring and ringing in the ears, sometimes changing into pleasant music. A persistent hissing noise in the ear, causing dizziness and a feeling of falling through the floor.
Sulphur	Extremely acute hearing, the least noise is unbearable, even the playing of a piano can induce nausea. Tinkling and roaring in the ears, but chiefly humming, usually at night in bed.

TIREDNESS *See* EXHAUSTION – PHYSICAL

TONSILLITIS

Chiefly affects children and young adults. The sore throat symptoms are made worse by swallowing, even liquids and saliva can cause acute discomfort. The voice becomes thick and breath becomes foul.

TREATMENT	*Aconite, Apis mel, Belladonna, Hepar Sulph, Lycopodium, Merc Sol, Phosphorus*
Aconite	Tonsils burning, smarting, dry and very red. High temperature with great thirst for cold water. Usually sudden onset at night, after exposure to cold raw wind.

Apis mel   Tonsils swollen, bright red, with stinging burning pain when swallowing which extends to the ears. Cluster of small blisters appear at the back of the throat.

Belladonna   Worse on the right side, bright red and burning hot, with the formation of small ulcers. The throbbing pain extends to the ear. Constant desire to swallow, which is painful and difficult.

Hepar Sulph   Chronic, with inflamed, swollen tonsils and neck glands. Inflammation of the tonsils, with the formation of an abscess, discharging a yellow pus. When swallowing there is a sensation like a splinter or fish bone in the throat. Hardness of hearing sometimes accompanies the symptoms.

Lycopodium   Chronic enlargement of the tonsils with swelling and suppuration, the pains moving from right to left. Tonsils pitted with small suppurating ulcers. They are worse from cold drinks, and frequently from 4 to 8pm

Merc Sol   Dryness of the throat with painful swallowing. Rawness, roughness and burning in the throat, but due to the excessive amount of saliva, frequent swallowing is unavoidable. Tonsils are dark red, studded with ulcers, accompanied by stinging pains and foul breath.

Phosphorus   Tonsils and the back of the throat swollen, dry, shining, painful, stinging and raw. Hawking of a heavy mucus, which is cold as it comes into the mouth and has a horrible taste.

TOOTHACHE
Usually caused by dental caries. The mouth and gums may be affected. Consult your dentist as soon as possible.

TREATMENT	*Aconite, Arnica, Belladonna, Chamomilla, Merc Sol*
Aconite	Brought on by cold, after exposure to cold winds, with throbbing in the left side of the face and intense redness of the cheek. Suitable for children where there is screaming with pain and restlessness.
Arnica	After extraction, with a tearing pain in all the teeth of the right upper jaw, extending to the ear. *Arnica* will stop the bleeding and promote healing of the gums.
Belladonna	Affecting the upper teeth on the right side, accompanied by much throbbing and a very hot red face. Toothache some minutes after eating but not during, increasing gradually to a high degree of pain and then gradually diminishing.
Chamomilla	Pains are severe and accompanied by heat, redness and swollen cheeks. Induced by taking anything warm into the mouth. A child may be peevish, and whine but is usually calmed down by petting.
Merc Sol	Pain ceases at night, but returns, in spasms, in the morning. Worse after either hot or cold drinks and relieved by rubbing the part of the cheek near the tooth.

TRAVEL SICKNESS *See* FIRST AID SECTION – SEA-SICKNESS

ULCERS
Of the skin.

TREATMENT	*Graphites, Hepar Sulph, Merc Sol, Sepia, Silica, Sulphur*
Graphites	Chronic ulcers with proud flesh, discharging a foul smelling pus and with itching and stinging pains. Sensitive, sore, spongy ulcers, oozing a thick sticky honey-like mucus

Hepar Sulph   Skin unhealthy, all slight injuries suppurate. Foul ulcers with sensitive edges surrounded by small blisters, burning, painful and discharging bloody pus.

Merc Sol   Generally burning, oozing a foul smelling pus at the edges. With hard, raised and jagged edges, painful and sensitive to touch and with a bluish-black colour.

Sepia   Itching, stinging and burning ulcers surrounded by blisters, frequently found on the heel or ankle. Painless ulcers on the joints or tips of the fingers or toes.

Silica   Unhealthy looking skin, every injury tends to ulcerate. Wherever pus is discharged or where ulcers are slow to develop and slow to heal. There is a sensation of coldness in the ulcer.

Sulphur   Unhealthy looking skin, the slightest injury is followed by burning inflammation and ulceration, usually surrounded by a bluish-red area. Ulcers are extremely itchy, burning and smarting.

URINE (DYSURIA)
Painful, slow and difficult urination.

TREATMENT   *Aconite, Apis mel, Belladonna, Cantharis, Nux vom*

Aconite   Urination painful and difficult, passed drop by drop and accompanied by great thirst, anxiety and restlessness.

Apis mel   Frequent desire to urinate, passing only a few drops of burning, stinging urine. Great intolerance of any form of heat and no thirst.

Belladonna   Painful burning and difficult discharge of blood and urine. Involuntary dribbling when standing or walking.

Cantharis	Acute urinary distress with straining and great frequency. Scalding and cutting pains before, during and after urination. The urge to urinate is worse when standing or walking and better when sitting. Painful dribbling, and a discharge sometimes mixed with blood.
Nux vom	Painful ineffectual urge to urinate, but can only pass a few drops. There is much straining, accompanied by painful burning.

URINE (INCONTINENCE OF)
BEDWETTING

TREATMENT	*Apis mel, Argent Nit, Belladonna, Pulsatilla, Sepia*
Apis mel	Involuntary discharge of painful and burning urine, chiefly at night in bed and worse from coughing. Intolerance of any form of heat and no thirst. Incontinence in old men where there is ·high coloured scanty discharge of smarting urine.
Argent Nit	Incontinence at night and also during the day. The urine burns while passing. The patient is very nervous and restless.
Belladonna	Constant urge to urinate. Dribbles urine during sleep. Involuntary dribbling when standing or walking. Starts in sleep and wets the bed.
Pulsatilla	Dribbling when standing, walking or coughing. Cannot retain urine, bedwetting at night especially in children and old people.
Sepia	Children and old people wet the bed as soon as they go to sleep. Have to rise frequently during the night to pass urine and always there is great urgency to do so.

URTICARIA *See* NETTLERASH

VARICOSE ULCERS
Ulceration of the leg, due to varicose veins or the result of an injury. **Get medical aid as soon as possible.**
See ULCERS

TREATMENT	*Carbo veg, Hamamelis, Merc Sol, Sulphur*
Carbo veg	Bluish varicose ulcers, bleeding easily with a scanty discharge of a foul smelling liquid. Tend to spread, slow to heal, accompanied by burning, especially at night. There is great weakness and coldness with poor circulation.
Hamamelis	Varicose ulcers with bruising and stinging pain. The bleeding causes acute exhaustion. Circulation is poor and the legs may be icy cold.
Merc Sol	With an extremely foul yellow discharge and which spread rapidly. There may be profuse nauseating sweat.
Sulphur	Varicose ulcers, sluggish with discharge and accumulation of greenish yellow pus. There is much itching with a tendency to become chronic.

VARICOSE VEINS
Enlarged, tortuous veins in the tissues under the skin of the leg. Rest the leg as much as possible and **get medical aid.**

TREATMENT	*Carbo veg, Hamamelis, Pulsatilla*
Carbo veg	Varicose veins, with blueness under the skin and burning pain. There may be bluish black patches due to poor circulation. Very chilly with cold feet, legs and knees.
Hamamelis	Varicose veins with purple blotches under the skin and congested veins accompanied by tiredness and painful leg muscles.
Pulsatilla	Inflamed varicose veins of the leg with much pain and poor circulation. The veins have a bluish colour and the pains are

stinging, usually more comfortable when walking about in cool air.

VERRUCA
A wart. A small abnormal growth on the skin.

TREATMENT	*Calc Carb, Natrum Mur, Sepia, Sulphur, Thuja*
Calc Carb	Skin unhealthy, many small warts especially on the sides of the fingers, the hands and arms.
Natrum Mur	Brown or black warts. Warts on the palms of the hands. Old warts on the nose and face.
Sepia	Large, hard, horny warts on the hands and fingers with deformed nails.
Sulphur	Skin dry, scaly and unhealthy with hard painful throbbing warts.
Thuja	Crops of warts on the back of the hand. Broad conical warts, flat black warts sometimes oozing moisture and bleeding. Warts on any part of the body.

VOICE, LOSS OF
See also LARYNGITIS

TREATMENT	*Argent Nit, Arnica, Belladonna, Carbo veg, Phosphorus*
Argent Nit	Chronic loss of voice of singers, raising the voice causes coughing.
Arnica	Hoarseness from over-use of the voice. The voice is deep and with a feeling of rawness in the wind pipe.
Belladonna	Burning dryness of the throat with hoarseness or complete loss of voice. Speech difficult and voice weak.
Carbo veg	Hoarseness and rawness of voice in the evening, painless loss of voice in the morning.

Phosphorus	Sensitiveness and dryness of the throat, cannot speak because of pain. Hoarseness and rawness in the throat, with tickling cough.

VOMITING

Commonly due to excessive eating, or emotional upset. **Get medical aid** if you vomit blood or black material, if you feel dizzy or have abdominal pain when vomiting.

TREATMENT	*Arsen Alb, Bryonia, Ipecac, Nux vom, Phosphorus*
Arsen Alb	Vomiting bitter watery fluid, after eating or drinking. Unquenchable burning thirst, drinks frequently, but only a little at a time.
Bryonia	Vomiting of solid food immediately after eating. Heartburn in the evening from wine. Nausea and vomiting in the morning when waking
Ipecac	Constant nausea, copious vomiting of sour fluid and mucus. Empty belching with copious saliva.
Nux vom	Heartburn and nausea early in the morning. Vomiting of food, liquid, bile and sour mucus after eating and from the effects of tobacco.
Phosphorus	Vomiting of food in mouthfuls until the stomach is empty. Great thirst for cold water and food, which as soon as they become warm in the stomach are ejected.

WARTS *See* VERRUCA

WHITLOW

A red, tender, suppurative infection in the folds of tissue surrounding the finger nail.

TREATMENT	*Apis mel, Belladonna, Graphites, Hepar Sulph, Silica*
Apis mel	Burning, stinging, throbbing of the tissue. It has a whitish appearance, is very painful, and the finger swells rapidly. Usually there is relief given by cold water.
Belladonna	Skin scarlet and smooth, greatly inflamed with burning, stinging and throbbing pain.
Graphites	Ulceration of the sides and roots of the finger nails. Exceedingly painful, burning and throbbing, then suppuration and proud flesh.
Hepar Sulph	Violent burning and throbbing of the fingers, with cutting pain at the root of the nail. Extremely tender to touch and sensitive to cold.
Silica	Violent shooting pain deep in the finger, worse from the warmth of the bed. Slow in developing and with a discharge of watery, greenish foul-smelling liquid.

WOUNDS *See* FIRST AID SECTION

WRY NECK

Stiff neck. A contracted state of the neck muscles producing twisting of the neck and an unnatural position of the head.

TREATMENT	*Aconite, Acatea rac, Belladonna, Bryonia, Lycopodium, Nux vom, Rhus tox*
Aconite	Painful stiff neck, pain extends down to the right shoulder. Sudden onset may be caused by exposure to cold draughts, or from a chill.
Actaea rac	Cramp in the neck muscles when moving the head. Stiff neck from exposure to cold air, pain on moving the hands.
Belladonna	Painful swelling and stiffness of the nape of the neck, worse on bending the head backwards.

Bryonia	Tearing pain in the muscles of the nape of the neck, so severe keeping still is impossible; however, the least movement makes the pain worse. Heat and pressure on the painful area gives relief.
Lycopodium	Tearing pain in the right side of the neck, extending downwards to the shoulder, arms and fingers.
Nux vom	Stiffness of the neck muscles especially after exposure to cold air or a draught of damp air.
Rhus tox	Stiff neck after getting wet or sleeping on damp ground. There is much tension and pain when moving accompanied by pain in the shoulders and the back.

At all times, if symptoms are serious or prolonged — contact your doctor as soon as possible.

Homoeopathic First Aid

Remember – If there is no improvement in the condition or injury after a short period you should call a qualified doctor for advice.

BITES AND STINGS
In all cases of bites and stings involving the mouth or throat, especially where there is great distress and difficulty in breathing – treat for shock and **get medical aid immediately**.

BEE STINGS
Remove the sting with tweezers. Cool the area with ice or a cold dressing.

TREATMENT	*Arnica, Urtica Urens Tincture*
Arnica	Where the wound feels bruised and is very painful to touch.
Urtica Urens Tincture (External Application)	If there is a stinging nettle type of rash around the sting, apply a compress of gauze saturated with a solution of *Urtica Urens Tincture* – two drops to one tablespoonful of water. One drop of *Urtica Urens Tincture* applied to the bee sting will prevent swelling.

WASP STINGS
Clean the area with lemon juice or vinegar. If in the mouth or throat take cold drinks, or suck ice cubes. If there is great distress, treat for shock and **get medical aid**.

TREATMENT	*Arnica*
Arnica	If the sting is painful to touch and feels bruised.

(External Application)	To prevent swelling apply one drop of *Arnica Tincture* to the sting.

HORSEFLIES, SANDFLIES, BED-BUGS, FLEAS AND MOSQUITOS
Clean the area with methylated spirit or surgical spirit. If distressed and anxious, treat for shock.

TREATMENT *Hypericum* (External Application)	*Hypericum* Where there is swelling with burning and stinging pain, affecting the nerves and pain shooting upwards. Apply one drop of *Hypericum Tincture* or *Ledum Tincture* to the bites.

NOTE A very useful protection from the treatment of minor bites and stings is a spray of Pyrethrum Compound.

ANIMAL BITES AND SCRATCHES
Clean the area with surgical spirit. In the case of deep wounds – treat for shock and **get medical aid**.

TREATMENT *Aconite*	*Aconite, Hypericum* In the case of deep wounds, for the shock, anxiety and fear, especially if the patient is extremely restless and inconsolable.
Hypericum (External Application)	For the stinging pain and injury to the nerves and pain which travels upwards. Apply one drop of *Hypericum Tincture* to the bite or scratch. In the case of deep wounds or bites, apply a compress of gauze saturated with a solution of *Hypericum Tincture*, two drops to one table-spoonful of water

BLACK EYE

TREATMENT	*Arnica, Ledum, Hamamelis Tincture*

Arnica	For sore bruised feeling around the eye, painful to touch and with much bluish red discolouration and unbroken skin.
Ledum	For painful hot swellings, especially if relieved by cold applications, suitable after taking *Arnica*.
Hamamelis Tincture (External Application)	Apply a compress of gauze saturated with a solution of *Hamamelis Tincture* – two drops to one tablespoonful of water.

BLISTERS
Avoid bursting the blister. If the blister does burst, cover the area with gauze and apply a compress of gauze saturated with a solution of *Urtica Urens Tincture*, two drops to one tablespoonful of water.

BRUISES

TREATMENT	*Arnica, Ruta grav*
Arnica	For the pain and shock from any mechanical injury, falls, blows or bruises.
Ruta grav	For the bruises and mechanical injury of bones, muscles and tendons.

NOTE Apply *Arnica Ointment* to most bruises, but if the skin is broken apply *Hypericum* and *Calendula Ointment*.

BURNS
Cool the affected area at once for several minutes with cold water. Remove rings, bracelets etc before swelling makes this difficult. Remove clothes if soaked in boiling fat, water, steam or chemicals. Wash chemical burns with cold running water. When in doubt treat for shock and **Get medical aid immediately**, especially for severe electric burns.

TREATMENT   *Cantharis*
Cantharis   For the burning pain before or after the
                   formation of blisters; the skin is red and
                   peeling.

NOTE For kitchen or cooking burns, rinse in cold water and
apply dressing of a homoeopathic *Burn Ointment*, cover with
gauze, lint or a bandage to keep the air out.

COLLAPSE
Fainting or a sudden loss of consciousness may be caused by
severe pain, sudden emotional shock, and can be made worse
by a hot stuffy room. Loosen any tight clothing, open
windows. Do not give anything to drink to a person who is
unconscious. If the patient does not come round in a few
minutes **get medical aid**.

TREATMENT   *Carbo veg*
Carbo veg   Crush one tablet very finely, place a small
                   portion inside the lips. Dissolve the
                   remainder in two tablespoonfuls of water.
                   Moisten the lips with this solution every
                   five minutes for one hour, or until help
                   arrives.

CUTS AND WOUNDS
Damage to the skin, and to the muscles if the wound is deep.
Clean the wound with surgical spirit, cover the wound to keep
clean. If the wound requires stitches, cover with a dry
dressing. **Get medical aid**.

TREATMENT   *Hypericum, Hypericum and Calendula*
                   Tincture
Hypericum   For injuries to nerves, especially fingers,
                   toes and toe nails, also for crushed
                   wounds, lacerated wounds and punctured
                   wounds.

| *(External Application)* | Apply a compress of gauze, saturated with a solution of *Hypericum and Calendula Tincture*, using two drops to one table-spoonful of water. If the cut is small apply one drop of *Hypericum and Calendula Tincture*. |

FRACTURES

Moving a person with a fracture requires skill. If in doubt do not touch the damaged area, or move the person, unless there is danger from fire, gas etc. **Get medical aid immediately**.

TREATMENT	*Arnica, Calc Phos*
Arnica	For the shock and bruising of all forms of mechanical injury, including fractures.
Calc Phos	For any type of fracture where there is slow union, or non-union, of the bones.

FRIGHT

TREATMENT	*Aconite, Gelsemium*
Aconite	A sudden most acute anxiety, a horrible fear leading to panic, intolerance and impatience.
Gelsemium	For the effects of sudden fright, bad or exciting news, or from the anticipation of some ordeal.

NOSE BLEED

When mild, it is due to the rupture of small blood vessels. Hold the soft part of the nose firmly between finger and thumb, lean head forward and hold nose for five or more minutes. If bleeding is severe **get medical aid immediately**.

| TREATMENT | *Ferrum Phos, Hamamelis, Phosphorus* |

Ferrum Phos	Nose bleed of bright red blood, especially in children. May be caused by injury, or a cold in the head.
Hamamelis	Profuse nose bleed with tightness of the bridge of the nose and with pressure in the forehead or between the eyes, which is relieved by the flow of blood.
Phosphorus	On blowing the nose and sneezing, with a profuse discharge of blood, often in the evening.

SCALDS
Burns caused by hot liquid or steam. *See* BURNS

SEASICKNESS, MOTION SICKNESS, TRAVEL SICKNESS
With a tendency to retching, nausea and vomiting. *See also* MORNING SICKNESS and NAUSEA – AILMENT SECTION

TREATMENT	*Arsen Alb, Ipecac, Nux vom*
Arsen Alb	Frequent excessive nausea, rising up to the throat, with an inclination to vomit. Frequently this is accompanied by an unquenchable thirst. Drinks often but only a little at a time.
Ipecac	With persistent vomiting, which does not relieve the nausea. This is accompanied by a copious flow of watery saliva and empty belching. The tongue remains clean.
Nux vom	Frequent nausea, and inclination to vomit. Nausea after a meal, with a flow back of food and liquid into the mouth. Nausea from tobacco smoke.

SHOCK

TREATMENT	*Aconite, Arnica, Carbo veg, Ignatia, Sepia*
Aconite	Great fear and anxiety after injury or from emotional upset, accompanied by fever, great restlessness and cannot be pacified.
Arnica	From injury, maybe accompanied by sickness and vomiting. The whole body feels sore and bruised, also general feeling of cold except for the head and face.
Carbo veg	After injury, emotional anxiety causes trembling. Chilly, with cold hands, ears and nose, cold knees and feet and even when shivering requires a window opened.
Ignatia	From anxiety, grief, bereavement, emotional stress and resentment. The excitement can cause painless diarrhoea.
Sepia	After the emotional shock has passed, and when resting, there is an outbreak of sweat. Becomes sad, silent, solitary, with a feeling of great apathy and indifference.

SPRAINS AND STRAINS

A SPRAIN is a joint injury with torn ligaments.
A STRAIN is an injury due to over-exercise or misuse of muscles.

TREATMENT	*Arnica, Rhus tox, Ruta grav*
Arnica	A feeling as if the joints of the arms and wrists were strained. Soreness after any type of muscular effort or sprain from a fall.
Rhus tox	For sprains after a fall or injury, with pain, stiffness and swelling. For sprains due to straining muscles or tendons by overlifting or stretching.
Ruta grav	Sprains of tendons, especially of the wrists, knuckles, knees and ankles, with or without swelling. Bones feel bruised and painful.

STINGS AND BITES *See* BITES AND STINGS

SUNBURN
Sunburn appears first as intense redness and tenderness of the exposed area. This may pass off quickly or it may increase, with the affected area blistering. *See also* BURNS AND SCALDS (FIRST AID SECTION)

TREATMENT   *Cantharis, Urtica Urens*
Cantharis   For burns before blisters form and when they have formed. Intense burning. There may be an urge to urinate.
Urtica Urens   For burns with intensive and persistent stinging.

If you have had too much sun and the skin is stinging, make a solution of *Urtica Urens Tincture*, using two drops to two tablespoonfuls of water. Apply frequently to the affected parts.

SUNSTROKE
HEAT EXHAUSTION, produced by exposure to the heat of the sun. There may be signs of prickly heat before the onset of exhaustion. There is fatigue during and after physical effort, even at rest. There is frontal headache, dizziness with blurred vision. The skin is cold and clammy, with profuse sweating on forehead and palms.

TREATMENT   *Aconite, Belladonna, Gelsemium, Natrum Mur, Pulsatilla*
Aconite   From sleeping in the sun. Sudden onset of fever, with burning of the head and face and with excessive thirst. Great fear and restlessness with dizziness and nausea. No matter how high the fever, *Aconite* is not indicated if the patient remains quiet.
Belladonna   Sudden onset of a rush of blood to the head with a throbbing headache. Red flushed

face, skin red and hot. Breathlessness, dizziness and restlessness with nausea and vomiting, accompanied by a rise of temperature and rapid pulse. Pupils dilated and eyes brilliant. The head may be hot with the hands and feet cold.

Gelsemium Depression from the heat of the sun. Headache from the neck over the head, with a bursting sensation in the forehead and eyeballs, with nausea and vomiting, cold sweat and cold feet. Irritable and excitable with dizziness as if intoxicated. Face flushed and hot to touch but there is no thirst.

Natrum Mur Face flushed and red, with nausea and vomiting. Hot weather causes fatigue, listlessness, dizziness and faintness. There is unquenchable thirst. Chronic one-sided headache, feels as if the head will burst.

Pulsatilla Throbbing headache with dizziness, nausea and loss of appetite. Irresistible desire for open air, but the heat of the sun is intolerable. Chilly yet worse for heat.

WOUNDS

Injuries to the body caused by physical means. *See* BITES AND STINGS, BRUISES, CUTS AND WOUNDS, SPRAINS AND STRAINS

TREATMENT *Arnica, Calendula, Hypericum*

Arnica For any injury, falls and bruises, fractures and effects of sprains and strain.

Calendula For an open wound make a solution of Calendula tincture, two drops to one teaspoonful of water. Clean the wound with this solution, saturate a gauze pad with the solution and cover the wound.

Hypericum For lacerated, punctured wounds, with torn tissue and involving the nerves. Crushed fingers, extremely painful, with the pain shooting up the limb. **Get medical aid**.

Homoeopathic Medicine Pictures

Study the Medicine Pictures carefully and select the medicine which most closely matches your symptoms.

You do not have to experience **all** the symptoms listed under a medicine nor need you exhibit **all** the likes or dislikes where mentioned; they are often expressed as an extreme which may not always apply. Simply try to match up with the set of symptoms most similar to those suffered.

ACONITE
Useful when taken at the onset of an illness, especially one brought on by an exposure to cold weather, colds and 'flu etc.

AILMENTS OR SYMPTOMS

Symptoms are sudden, violent and brief
Exposure to draughts or a cold wind
Dry suffocating cough
Sore throat following exposure to cold, dry winds
High temperature with great thirst
Great pain
Bereavement, grief, anxiety, restlessness, fear
Animal bites
Sleeplessness
Intolerance of pain
Stiff neck
Tinnitus
Tonsillitis
Teething and toothache
Liverish
Periods suppressed or delayed due to worry or fear

SYMPTOMS WORSEN	At midnight
	When lying on affected side
	In a warm room
	From tobacco smoke
	In cold winds
	Listening to music

| SYMPTOMS IMPROVE | In the open air |
| | With the bedclothes thrown off |

ACTAEA RAC

AILMENTS OR SYMPTOMS	Neuralgia
	Stiff neck
	Painful muscles following strenuous exercise
	Shooting pains
	Heavy periods
	Rheumatic pains in back and neck

| SYMPTOMS WORSEN | In cold and damp |
| | When moving |

SYMPTOMS IMPROVE	In warmth
	When eating
	Headaches improve in the open air

APIS MEL

Helpful in the treatment of burning or stinging pains where flushed swelling or puffing is present. It is especially good for swelling of the lower eyelid. Symptoms are mostly on the right side.

AILMENTS OR SYMPTOMS	Effects of insect stings
	Burning stinging pains
	Swelling of lower eyelids

Absence of thirst
Synovitis
Listlessness, lack of concentration
Swollen gums
Incontinence in old people
Itching
Nettlerash
Shingles
Teething
Sore throat
Tonsillitis
Whitlow

SYMPTOMS WORSEN	From getting wet During late afternoon After sleeping From heat in any form When touched When in a closed and heated room
SYMPTOMS IMPROVE	From a change of position or walking about In the open air From cold bathing

ARGENT NIT

A good medicine for anxiety, apprehension or fear. Useful when taken before any difficult undertaking – making a speech etc.

AILMENTS OR SYMPTOMS	Acidity, heartburn Craving for sweet food, cheese, fats or salt followed by upset stomach with much wind Dizziness from overwork and mental strain Itching scalp Irregular blotches on skin

SYMPTOMS WORSEN	From warmth in any form Craves cold air After eating sweet foods From over-work Worry about the future
SYMPTOMS IMPROVE	From belching Cold, fresh air

ARNICA

Especially suited to complaints which have been caused by any injury, however remote. Can also be taken in cases of mental or physical shock.

AILMENTS OR SYMPTOMS	Use after any injury – lessens shock Bruises Sprains Physical exhaustion following sustained exercise, eg a day's gardening or a long walk Sleeplessness due to over-tiredness Muscles ache all over Bed feels too hard – constant desire to move over to a soft part Gout, rheumatism with a fear of being touched Aids recovery after an operation or childbirth Loss of voice Toothache Bee and wasp stings
SYMPTOMS WORSEN	From touch From exposure to hot sun From touch From motion In damp cold conditions

| SYMPTOMS IMPROVE | When lying down, with head low |

ARSEN ALB
Beneficial when dealing with vomiting and diarrhoea caused by eating bad meat, fruit or vegetables.

| AILMENTS OR SYMPTOMS | Restlessness
Anxiety and great fear
Burning pains
Throat dry and burning
Burning pain in the stomach
Excessive thirst but with only the desire to sip a little and often
Food poisoning with vomiting and diarrhoea
Cannot bear the sight or smell of food
Psoriasis
Thrush
Carbuncle
Catarrh
Hayfever |

| SYMPTOMS WORSEN | After midnight up to 2–3am
Between 1–2pm
At the coast
From cold wet weather |

| SYMPTOMS IMPROVE | By keeping warm, with cool air round the head
From warm or hot drinks |

BELLADONNA
Always associated with red, hot skin; throbbing headaches, earaches and boils will benefit from this medicine. A very good remedy for children. Symptoms are usually severe and the onset is sudden.

AILMENTS OR SYMPTOMS	Brightly flushed face
	Swollen glands
	Swollen joints
	Boils
	Facial neuralgia
	Severe throbbing earache
	Chicken pox
	Sunstroke
	Throbbing headache
	Measles
	Air sickness
	Periods – early and profuse
	Mumps
	Rupture
	Cystitis
	Quinsy
	Whitlow
	Sore throat, tonsillitis
	Loss of voice
	Toothache and teething
	Wry neck
	Incontinence

SYMPTOMS WORSEN	In the afternoon and at night
	From noise
	From bright light
	From touch
	When lying down

SYMPTOMS IMPROVE	From warmth
	While sitting erect

BRYONIA

Can be used when there are stitching, tearing pains which are
worse from moving and better when resting.

AILMENTS OR SYMPTOMS	Chestiness – colds often go down into the chest
	Dryness of the air passages
	Dry painful cough, often violent
	Dry lips, tongue and throat
	Excessive thirst, especially cold drinks
	Food lies heavily in the stomach which is too painful to touch
	Lumbago
	Bronchitis
	Painful knee joint
	Painful hip joint
	Diarrhoea after eating over-ripe fruit, or drinking cold water when one is over-heated
	Rheumatism
	Gout
	Wry neck
SYMPTOMS WORSEN	From any movement
	From warmth

CALC CARB

AILMENTS OR SYMPTOMS	Overweight, especially in children and young persons
	Dislikes milk, coffee, tobacco and hot food
	Craving for eggs, wine, salt or sweet things
	Tendency to feel the cold and catch cold easily
	Cold damp feet and clammy hands
	Cracked skin
	Premenstrual tension
	Verruca

SYMPTOMS WORSEN	From cold air and draughts
	In damp weather
	At night
	From standing

SYMPTOMS IMPROVE	In dry weather
	From warmth (avoid the sun)
	While lying on the painful side

CALC FLUOR

| AILMENTS OR SYMPTOMS | Scars |

| SYMPTOMS WORSEN | After rest |
| | From damp, humid weather |

SYMPTOMS IMPROVE	After a little movement
	From warm applications
	Taking warm drinks

CALC PHOS
Fractures which are slow or difficult to heal can benefit from this medicine.

AILMENTS OR SYMPTOMS	Severe stomach pain after eating
	Fractures slow to heal
	Premenstrual pain with cramp
	Cold hands and feet

| SYMPTOMS WORSEN | From any change in the weather |
| | Cold wet weather and melting snow |

| SYMPTOMS IMPROVE | In dry warm weather |
| | From a hot bath |

CANTHARIS

Good for local irritations with raw, burning pains. A constant and intolerable urge to urinate is most common.

AILMENTS OR SYMPTOMS	Burning pains
	Burns and scalds before blisters form
	Sunburn
	Burning pain in the bladder before, during and after passing urine
	Cystitis
	Urine scalds and is passed drop by drop
	Constant urge to pass urine
SYMPTOMS WORSEN	From touch
	While passing urine
	After drinking cold water or coffee
SYMPTOMS IMPROVE	After belching or passing wind

CARBO VEG

Useful medicine for mild food poisoning when caused by fish.

AILMENTS OR SYMPTOMS	Heartburn with excessive wind
	Mild food poisoning after eating tainted fish
	Ailments following cold damp weather
	Varicose veins and ulcers
	Chilly but likes window open
	Hoarseness, rough throat without pain
	Loss of voice
SYMPTOMS WORSEN	After eating fatty foods
	During damp weather
	In the evening and at night
	In cold, frosty weather

SYMPTOMS IMPROVE	On bringing up wind
	By being fanned
	After sleep

CUPRUM MET
Useful in the treatment of cramps, especially when they start in the fingers and toes and spread.

AILMENTS OR SYMPTOMS	Night sweats and cramp in fingers, legs or toes
	Violent spasms and cramps
	Excessively chilly, yet thirsty for cold water

SYMPTOMS WORSEN	In the evening and at night
	In cold air and cold wind
	After vomiting which may be relieved by a drink of cold water

| SYMPTOMS IMPROVE | After a cold drink |
| | While sweating |

DROSERA
Helpful in the treatment of dry, spasmodic coughs.

AILMENTS OR SYMPTOMS	Always too cold, chilly even in bed
	Any cough with sudden violent attacks which may end in vomiting
	Deep hoarse barking cough with retching
	Constant tickling cough
	Laryngitis with a dry throat making it an effort to talk, exciting a cough with yellow mucus
	Sensation of having a feather in the throat
	Shivering when resting – no shivering when moving

SYMPTOMS WORSEN	From warmth
	After drinking
	While laughing
	When lying down
	After midnight

SYMPTOMS IMPROVE	In the open air and when walking

EUPHRASIA

Any watering or inflammation of the eyes and also a runny nose can benefit from this medicine.

AILMENTS OR SYMPTOMS	Colds with watering eyes and streaming nose
	Inflamed eyes which sting and burn
	Conjunctivitis
	Unable to tolerate bright light
	Hayfever
	First stage of measles
	Cough, better at night in bed

SYMPTOMS WORSEN	Indoors
	In the evening
	In bed
	During the night and morning
	From warmth and bright light

SYMPTOMS IMPROVE	In dim light or darkness
	From cold applications
	Getting out of bed
	From coffee and from eating

FERR PHOS

AILMENTS OR SYMPTOMS	Dizziness from congestion of the head
	Nosebleeds
	Suitable for first stage of acute inflammation and early colds, especially when without very definite symptoms
	Appetite varies greatly from insatiable hunger to total loss of appetite
	Excitable and talkative
	Headache with hot red face and vomiting food, cannot tolerate hair being touched; relieved by nosebleed
SYMPTOMS WORSEN	At night
	From cold
	From touch
SYMPTOMS IMPROVE	In summer
	From warmth
	From cold applications
	While slowly walking around

GELSEMIUM

Good in the treatment of influenza and influenza-like colds. It is also useful for the treatment of nervous apprehension, eg pre-examination nerves.

AILMENTS OR SYMPTOMS	Influenza
	Sneezing
	Sore throat
	Symptoms of flushing, aching, trembling
	Headache, throbbing, spreads from the nape of the neck to the forehead above the eyes, feel as if bound by a tight band
	Heavy eyes
	Trembling and weakness especially about the knees with a tendency to go cold

with an empty feeling, relieved by moving about

Weary with heavy aching muscles

Absence of thirst even with a high temperature

Difficulty in swallowing

Runny nose

Dizziness

Fear before an examination, before a driving test or going to school

Mental exhaustion

Writer's cramp

Neuralgia

Sunstroke

SYMPTOMS WORSEN	From sudden fright
	Undue excitement
	Bad news, vexation and anticipation
	When exposed to direct sunlight in a hot room
	Before a thunderstorm
	In cold damp weather
	Around 10am
	Movement aggravates most symptoms, but relieves muscular pains
SYMPTOMS IMPROVE	In the open air
	From continued movement
	From alcoholic stimulants
	After sweating
	After passing a large amount of pale urine

GRAPHITES

AILMENTS OR SYMPTOMS	Unhealthy looking skin
	Eczema with discharge of sticky fluid
	Tendency for injuries to suppurate
	Cracked finger tips and toes

Tinnitus, hears better when surrounded by noise

Whitlow

Psoriasis

Dry scabs in nose with sore cracked and ulcerated nostrils

Styes

Hot flushes

Premenstrual tension

SYMPTOMS WORSEN	At night, before midnight
	During and immediately after periods
	In draughts
	Cold and damp in all forms
	From heat of the bed or from exertion

SYMPTOMS IMPROVE	Resting in the dark
	From wrapping up but must have plenty of air

HAMAMELIS

Especially successful in the treatment of varicose veins and haemorrhoids.

AILMENTS OR SYMPTOMS	Varicose veins and ulcers
	Nosebleeds clear the head
	Piles which ooze dark blood
	Tired feeling in arms and legs with painful muscles and joints
	Bruised soreness of affected parts
	Chilblains, always with a bluish colour
	Black eye

SYMPTOMS WORSEN	During the day and when at rest but entirely absent at night
	From touch
	In warm moist air
	In a warm room

| SYMPTOMS
IMPROVE | In the open air
During periods of concentration |

HEPAR SULPH

Especially useful for injuries that tend to suppurate and are very sensitive to touch.

AILMENTS OR SYMPTOMS	Skin is generally unhealthy, moist and intensely sensitive to touch, even bandages and clothing on affected areas are very painful Injuries tend to suppurate Intense chilliness, sensitive to the least draught Croupy cough brought on by the least exposure to the cold air, with rattling in chest but no expectoration Quinsy Wheezing Sensation of a splinter or fishbone at the back of the throat Earache with offensive discharge Chronic tonsillitis especially when accompanied by loss of hearing Whitlow Sinusitis
SYMPTOMS WORSEN	In cold air, cold dry winds and draughts When lying on painful side On uncovering the head When the affected parts are touched In the winter On awakening In the evening, after midnight
SYMPTOMS IMPROVE	From warmth From wrapping up especially the head After a meal In warm wet weather

HYPERICUM

Very useful when treating injuries to the nerves, especially the fingers and toes as well as punctured wounds where the pain shoots up the limb. Excessive pain is a guiding symptom of this remedy.

AILMENTS OR SYMPTOMS	Wounds caused by sharp objects and by cat bites Very painful cuts and wounds involving nerve endings Falls injuring spine Headache with a floating sensation as a result of a fall Blows on fingers or toes Horse-fly bites
SYMPTOMS WORSEN	From the cold and damp, especially in fog and before a storm From touch From 6pm to 10pm In the dark
SYMPTOMS IMPROVE	While bending head backwards When keeping still

IGNATIA

One of the chief medicines for hysteria; very useful when dealing with effects of grief or worry.

AILMENTS OR SYMPTOMS	Shock Fright and changeable moods Prolonged, silent, pent-up grief Dislike of tobacco smoke Throbbing headache Sciatica

SYMPTOMS WORSEN	In the morning
	From cold
	Eating sweets, coffee or alcohol
	From tobacco smoke

| SYMPTOMS IMPROVE | While eating |
| | From a change of position |

IPECAC

The principal symptoms which benefit from this medicine are persistent nausea and vomiting.

| AILMENTS OR SYMPTOMS | Any illness where there is constant nausea and sickness – Morning sickness, Travel sickness |
| | Bronchitis |

SYMPTOMS WORSEN	Periodically
	When lying down
	In cold weather
	After eating veal or pork

SYMPTOMS IMPROVE	When at rest
	With the eyes closed
	In the open

KALI BICH

AILMENTS OR SYMPTOMS	Complaints brought on by a change to hot weather
	Catarrh with a stringy discharge
	Sinusitis
	Sore throat
	Migraine – blurred vision before headache
	Pains move rapidly

SYMPTOMS WORSEN	In the morning, especially 2am–5am
	From alcohol
	During hot weather
	Sudden onset of hot weather can aggravate rheumatic conditions

| SYMPTOMS IMPROVE | From heat, especially when tucked up in a warm bed |

KALI PHOS

Excellent nerve remedies, especially for young people. Any complaints arising from a lack of mental energy or involving mental or physical depression will benefit greatly from this remedy. Symptoms are often caused by excitement, overwork and worry.

AILMENTS OR SYMPTOMS	Mental exhaustion from overwork
	Nervous exhaustion
	Exhaustion following long periods of preparation for exams

| SYMPTOMS WORSEN | From noise, excitement and worry |
| | From mental and physical exertion |

SYMPTOMS IMPROVE	During gentle movement
	From warmth
	After nourishment

LYCOPODIUM

AILMENTS OR SYMPTOMS	Abdominal pain
	Dislike of exercise
	Anticipatory fear of failure
	Preference to be alone (but with somebody near)
	Excessive hunger even at night which is easily satisfied
	Heartburn, craving for sweet foods even though they cause indigestion

Coldness in one foot while the other is warm

Pains moving from left to right

Cystitis – passing large quantities of pale urine, which sometimes contains a red sand or brick dust-like sediment

Premenstrual tensions and irritability relieved when period starts

Hiccough with acidity and bloated abdomen

Nettlerash

Tinnitus

Wry neck

Rupture

Tonsillitis

SYMPTOMS WORSEN	Between 4pm–8pm
	Better in the morning but bad tempered on waking
	In stuffy rooms
	From cold air, cold food or liquid
	When occupied, hurried or worried

SYMPTOMS IMPROVE	After warm drinks
	On loosening clothing around the abdomen
	In cold, fresh air
	Active occupation gives relief

MERC SOL

AILMENTS OR SYMPTOMS	Profuse offensive sweating
	Sore throat with excessive foul saliva
	Swollen tongue flabby and indented, moist with great thirst
	Tonsillitis
	Mumps
	Suppuration of injuries
	Varicose veins and ulcers
	Slimy, metallic taste in the mouth
	Greyish mouth ulcers

Thrush (mouth)
Intense thirst
Toothache at night, worse from either hot
or cold fluid

SYMPTOMS   At night
WORSEN   In a warm room
                  From heat and from cold
                  During wet or changeable weather

SYMPTOMS   When resting in bed
IMPROVE   When at high altitudes

NATRUM MUR

AILMENTS OR   Sneezy colds
SYMPTOMS   Nose runs like a tap (treat quickly at onset)
                   Sinusitus
                   Very sensitive, likes to be left alone
                   Verruca
                   Cold sores (herpes), upper lip swollen,
                       crack in the middle of lower lip
                   Thrush (mouth) with ulcers on tongue
                   Nettlerash with large red blotches, itchy,
                       burning and smarting
                   Menstrual pain when both sad and irritable
                   Premenstrual tension with weeping and
                       laughing
                   Migraine with paleness, nausea and
                       vomiting
                   Coldness of knees, down the legs to the feet
                   Continuous thirst, especially for tea
                   Dislike of bread, meat and coffee
                   Copious use of salt on food
                   Exhaustion from trifling cause, with sensa-
                       tion of throbbing all over, frequently
                       worse in the morning
                   Sunstroke

SYMPTOMS WORSEN	In mid-morning
	Near the coast – sometimes better
	From extremes of temperature
	From hot sun, radiant heat, heat of a fire
	Warm stuffy atmosphere
	While lying down

SYMPTOMS IMPROVE	In the open air
	On bright sunny days
	While lying on the right side
	While cold bathing
	After a sweat
	When fasting

NUX VOM

Very successful when dealing with the bad effects of alcohol, tobacco, coffee and over-eating.

AILMENTS OR SYMPTOMS	Tense, over-anxious and jittery
	Heartburn two to three hours after eating
	Morning sickness
	Sleeplessness
	Abdominal pain
	Over-sensitive to noise, odours, light, music
	Ill effects of over-eating or drinking
	Early morning liverishness from alcoholic excess
	Travel sickness, acid vomiting from least motion
	Fussiness about food, liking for fatty foods
	Dislike of coffee and tobacco smoke
	Burning and itching piles
	Stuffy colds
	Painful ineffectual urge to urinate
	Wry neck
	Rupture

| SYMPTOMS WORSEN | Between 3am–4am or after waking in the morning |
| | From cold, dry, windy weather |

| SYMPTOMS IMPROVE | In the evening from being covered |
| | From warmth and uninterrupted sleep |

PHOSPHORUS

AILMENTS OR SYMPTOMS	Bronchitis with dry cough, soreness and rawness in the air passages and discharge of sticky mucus
	Cough hard and dry from a persistent tickle
	Hoarseness, laryngitis, loss of voice
	Craving for cold food and drink (eg ices and cold water) which is vomited once warmed in the stomach
	Vomiting
	Tinnitus
	Tonsillitis
	Fear of darkness or thunderstorms
	Recurrent styes
	Small wounds with a tendency to bleed easily

SYMPTOMS WORSEN	In the evening
	From putting hands in cold water
	While lying on the left side
	After warm food and drink

| SYMPTOMS IMPROVE | While lying on the right side or on the back in a warm room and when warmly covered |
| | Open air relieves headache |

PULSATILLA

The patients' disposition and mental state are the guiding symptoms for this medicine. It is predominantly a remedy for

women and is successful when treating persons of affec-
tionate, mild and yielding character who are often prone to
weepiness.

AILMENTS OR
SYMPTOMS
	Catarrh (yellow-green thick discharge)
	Hayfever
	Styes on the margin of the lids
	Conjunctivitis and thick yellow discharge
	Mumps with swelling of the glands
	Measles with dry or loose cough and
	    intolerance of light
	Menopause
	Loneliness
	Sinusitis
	Varicose veins
	Incontinence
	Menstrual pain, griping with nausea and
	    vomiting
	Premenstrual tension, weepy, sad and pale
	    faced
	Periods – suppressed, delayed or irregular
	Cystitis with frequency, pain and distress
	Inflammation with swelling or redness
	    shifting rapidly from joint to joint
	Rapid change in symptoms – from feeling
	    well to feeling miserable
	Pains shifting and variable
	Aversion to fat or greasy food
	Absence of thirst (even in fever) though
	    the mouth may be dry

SYMPTOMS WORSEN	In the evening before midnight From heat, close atmosphere, humidity After eating rich foods From sudden chilling when hot
SYMPTOMS IMPROVE	In the open air, especially cold, dry air From cold applications and after cold food and drinks While lying on the painful side From uncovering

RHUS TOX

For complaints associated with sprains and strains of joints or tendons, caused by over-exertion. It is also useful when treating toxic conditions resulting in rashes.

AILMENTS OR SYMPTOMS	Effects of over-exertion, strain, operations etc
	Strains of joints or tendons
	Rheumatism, lumbago, sciatica
	Pain in ligaments
	Chicken pox, itchy and burning at night
	Shingles
	Eczema
	Gout
	Cold sores (Herpes Simplex) of mouth and nose
	Chilblains, burning itchy and blotchy, after scratching there may be spots with pus
	Thirst
	Tickling cough
	Tongue with red triangular tip
	Acute anxiety, fear, restlessness
	Synovitis
	Wry neck
SYMPTOMS WORSEN	On beginning to move
	From cold and wet
	During rest
	After midnight
	Pain increases on beginning to move but tends to diminish if a gentle movement is maintained
SYMPTOMS IMPROVE	During warm weather
	With gentle movement
	From warm applications

RUTA GRAV

Any bruising or fracture of a small bone will be helped by this medicine.

AILMENTS OR SYMPTOMS	Injuries to bones – bruised bones, fractures, dislocations
	Sprains of wrists and ankles
	Pains as if bruised. Tennis elbow
	Rheumatism with pain in tendons and muscles
	Eye strain – eyes burning and aching
	Synovitis, inflammation of the larger joints especially of the upper extremities

SYMPTOMS WORSEN	From cold and during wet weather
	While lying down on the painful part
	Walking out of doors
	Reading and straining the eyes

SYMPTOMS IMPROVE	From warmth and moving about indoors

SEPIA

AILMENTS OR SYMPTOMS	Indifference to loved ones
	Sadness and fear of being left alone
	Yellowness – especially of the face, with a saddle across the nose
	Sensation of faintness in the middle of the morning
	Incontinence
	Ulcers
	Verruca
	Sensitivity to cold air
	Premenstrual tension with colic
	Periods suppressed or delayed
	Menopause, sudden hot flushes with tendency to faint
	Hot sweats from the slightest exertion

SYMPTOMS WORSEN	In the afternoon and evening
	From cold

From consolation
Before thunder and from tobacco smoke

SYMPTOMS   In a warm bed
IMPROVE   From hot applications

SILICA

AILMENTS OR   Physical and mental debility due to over-
SYMPTOMS   exertion of the body or mind
                  Boils, carbuncles, abscesses, acne
                  Bunions
                  Whitlow
                  Helps the expulsion of foreign bodies eg
                      thorns and splinters
                  Styes
                  Ulcers
                  Suppuration
                  Quinsy
                  Sinusitis
                  Migraine, violent, periodic right-sided
                      headache

SYMPTOMS   From cold
WORSEN   In cold wet weather
                  From being uncovered
                  In approaching winter

SYMPTOMS   When warmly wrapped up
IMPROVE   Hot applications
                  In summer

SULPHUR
AILMENTS OR   Unhealthy looking skin, dry, rough, scaly
SYMPTOMS   and itchy
                  Tendency to skin diseases

Eczema

Psoriasis

Itching skin – scratching pleasurable but results in burning and itching

Piles, burning and itching; protrude, ooze and bleed

Nettlerash

Tendency to sweat, seldom offensive and at times cold

Varicose ulcers

Verruca

Openings of the body become bright red, eyelids, nostrils and anus

Burning pains

Burning soles of feet must be placed outside the bedclothes to cool

Sleeplessness, drowsy by day, wakefulness by night

Tinnitus, tinkling and humming, sometimes roaring and crackling in the ears or in the head

Mid-morning hunger

Large appetite for highly seasoned, spicy, fatty foods and sweets

Aggravation from milk, sweets and alcohol

Lack of energy (regained quickly at the prospect of pleasurable activity)

Tendency to become exhausted quickly, perhaps fainting

Tendency to catch cold easily which often goes into the chest

Thrush (of the mouth)

SYMPTOMS WORSEN	From heat, especially heat of the bed At night in bed Cold wet weather and severe cold
SYMPTOMS IMPROVE	From dry, not too hot weather In the morning

Motion relieves pains in the head and knees

THUJA
Very successful for treating warty growths.

AILMENTS OR SYMPTOMS	Warty growths on any part of the body
	Severe left frontal headache in the morning on waking and sometimes at bedtime, aggravated by sleeping
	Frequency of urine with acute cutting pain at the end of passing urine
	Sweat, only on uncovered parts, sweat is strong smelling and sweetish
	Verruca
	Sleeplessness
SYMPTOMS WORSEN	From cold, damp weather
	At night from the heat of the bed
	At 3am, after breakfast and 3pm
SYMPTOMS IMPROVE	After sweating
	From scratching or being massaged
	After stretching the limbs
	Rheumatic pains relieved in cool air

Medicines and Their Indications for Children's Ailments

Although in general the symptoms exhibited by adults and children should be treated in the same way, there are certain conditions and reactions that are peculiar to childhood. These can often be treated successfully by following the indications and medicines suggested in this section.

ACONITE
For the child who catches cold on getting wet. Child may be alert and alarmed, there may be piteous wailing. Hot, dry skin. Feverish thirst for cold water. Restless tossing at night. Give this medicine in the early stages before the condition becomes well established.

APIS MEL
This child is tearful and fidgety with retention of urine in nursing infants. Shrill, sudden piercing screams while sleeping or waking.

ARGENT NIT
Usually agitated and fidgety, with an irresistible desire for sweets and sugar; this causes sickness and vomiting of mouthfuls of liquid and greenish diarrhoea.

ARNICA
This is a most useful medicine for dealing with the bumps and bruises of childhood. It is especially helpful if the child is shocked after some little mishap. Arnica ointment applied externally is also helpful in clearing up a bruised surface. The medicine can be given before and after visiting the dentist to assist the natural healing process, especially after extractions.

ARSEN ALB

For the child who is over-tired and irritable even after the least exertion. Tummy pains from eating fruit, especially melon, also rich and oily foods; mild food poisoning. The child is restless and peevish, wants to go from person to person and to be carried quickly. Very thirsty, drinks often, but only a little at a time.

BELLADONNA

This child experiences sudden attacks of symptoms which usually include hot and red skin with flushed face and dilated pupils. Attacks are often violent and there may be great excitement with vomiting or severe headache. Use if the child has taken too much sun.

BRYONIA

In contrast to Belladonna, symptoms usually come on gradually. The child may be irritable and dislike being lifted or carried. Hard, dry cough with stitching pains in the chest, made worse by movement. Excessive thirst. Diarrhoea from sour fruit or from drinking cold water and getting overheated.

CALC PHOS

For pale-faced, thin, lanky children. The infant wants to suckle all the time and vomits easily. Children develop headache from watching television.

CANTHARIS

There is a constant urge to pass urine but the child usually cries from the pain. Mouth and throat may appear red and inflamed and liquids are swallowed with difficulty. Give when the mouth is burned from taking food which is too hot.

CHAMOMILLA (GRANULES)

This is for teething infants, intolerably peevish and irritable, extremely impatient and restless, best given in granule form. The child whines and is only pacified with constant petting.

DROSERA

May be used where the child has rapidly recurring fits of

coughing. There is choking, with great difficulty in breathing and possibly retching and vomiting.

GELSEMIUM
There is fear of the dark and fear of falling, the child grasps nurse or the side of the cot and screams with fear of falling. Influenza symptoms of shivering with cold, which may alternate with heat; aching all over. Diarrhoea from emotional excitement. Examination 'fears' in older children.

HEPAR SULPH
This child is over-sensitive and easily takes offence at the slightest thing. A very chilly child who must keep warm although he will easily perspire. Useful with splinter-like pains, especially the sensation of a bone stuck in the throat. Unhealthy skin, cuts and grazes tend to suppurate.

HYPERICUM
Use this remedy if the child jams its fingers in the door: it helps healing and relieves pain. If bitten or scratched by an animal and the pain travels upwards, always give a few doses and **get medical aid**. *Arnica* can also be given to control shock.

IPECAC
Diarrhoea of infants, with grass green, slimy stools. All complaints are accompanied by nausea and frequently shivering and yawning. The onset is sudden and progresses rapidly. The child passes copious amounts of greenish slime. In fat, pale children there is nausea, vomiting and colic with diarrhoea. The child wails and screams continuously.

LYCOPODIUM
Child awakens cross and angry, inclined to strike, bite, scratch and kick everyone who approaches. Painful urging to urinate, the child cries and grasps abdomen. There is a red sand deposit in the diaper and a rash where urine has inflamed the skin. Look out for the right foot being cold and left foot being of normal temperature.

MERC SOL

Violent toothache at night, followed by chilliness over the whole body. The child must always be taken to the dentist. For bad breath and where the child complains of a nasty taste in the mouth. Swollen neck glands and mouth ulcers.

NUX VOM

This child is fiery, excitable and irritable; is always chilly, hugs the fire. Cold in the head, and shivering, running nose during the day, dry at night. Loves a party, eats too much highly seasoned and rich food which may be followed by sourness of the mouth, retching and gagging. Vomiting is distressing and difficult, but gives relief. Tummy pains may be followed by constipation with frequent urging and scanty results.

PHOSPHORUS

For the delicate, sensitive, restless and excitable child, easily startled. Has nosebleeds of bright red blood and bleeds easily after tooth extraction or injury. Craves cold food, especially ice cold drinks, which are vomited as soon as they become warm in the stomach; vomiting is followed by violent thirst. Hard dry cough from a persistent tickle in the throat or low down behind the breast bone; worse talking or laughing and from cold air.

PULSATILLA

This child can be sad, obstinate, silent and peevish. Also for the child with a mild, gentle, yielding disposition, easily moved to tears. Fears the dark and ghosts. Likes to be fussed over and caressed. Useful for styes, measles and chilblains which are unbearable when hot. If the child fits this description of temperament use the remedy first no matter the ailment.

RHUS TOX

This is for the child who plays out in the rain and complains the next day of pains. May feel better after movement. These symptoms may also result from a lengthy visit to the swimming baths. Complaints come on before or during cold, wet weather.

SILICA
Weak puny child, eats plenty but assimilation is poor. Is constantly restless, self-willed, touchy and contrary. Unable to take any form of milk and the mother's milk causes diarrhoea and vomiting. The child is chilly even in a warm room, but there may be smelly night sweats. Sometimes there is bed wetting, with a yellow sand deposit in the diaper.

SULPHUR
This child is difficult to calm, cannot get what it wants quickly enough, becomes sulky and will not speak. Warm, hungry babies, kick off the bedclothes, impossible to keep them covered at night. Extreme brilliant redness of the lips, eyelids, nostrils and anus. Child cannot bear to be washed. Skin rough, scaly and very itchy.

Veterinary Homoeopathy

Animals in general respond well to Homoeopathy. Homoeopathic treatment is used effectively for domestic pets, including cats, dogs, rabbits, tortoises, birds, hamsters and guinea pigs. It is not surprising, for this system of healing has long been recognised as extremely effective in the treatment of human beings. Furthermore, homoeopathy has been proven, by long use, an alternative to conventional medicine.

Some people have tried to explain Homoeopathy's success by suggesting that its effectiveness depends on the psychology of the patient, that people believe they are going to be cured and so their minds condition their bodies to respond.

This obviously cannot be true of animals. Neither can an animal assist the vet by detailing how it feels. Diagnosis must be made on the basis of observation of the practitioner and by the owner. A caring owner will usually come to know an animal's temperament and habits and will notice if, for example, it shows fear under certain conditions, has a preference for the warmth or cold, or reacts in a distinctive way to strangers or other animals. All such information is important in deciding on the necessary treatment.

Given that an owner knows an animal well, it is perfectly feasible for minor ailments and conditions to be cleared up safely and simply at home using one or other of the homoeopathic remedies now available. See Veterinary Section in the list of Recommended Reading (Pages 117–118).

Glossary of Terms in Common Use

ACUTE
: An illness which lasts a short time and with pronounced symptoms.

AGGRAVATION
: A temporary worsening of symptoms which may occur during homoeopathic treatment as the remedy brings the infection to the surface whereupon it can be tackled and overcome more easily by the body's natural healing forces.

ALLOPATHY
: A word first used by Dr Samuel Hahnemann to describe the ordinary system of medical treatment.

CENTESIMAL
: The dilution of one part of substance to ninety nine parts of diluent. Homoeopathic medicines prepared on this scale are referred to as c or ch.

CHRONIC
: An illness persisting over a long period of time. The symptoms are constantly present or recur frequently.

CLASSICAL
: Traditional homoeopathy according to the principles established by Dr Samuel Hahnemann.

CONSTITUTIONAL MEDICINE
: A medicine prescribed on the basis of character, temperament and general reactions, as well as for the symptoms of the illness.

DECIMAL
: The dilution of one part of substance to nine parts of diluent. Homoeopathic medicines prepared on this scale are referred to as D or x.

HAHNEMANN
: Dr Christian Friedrich Samuel Hahnemann was born in Meissen, 10 April 1755. A brilliant student, Hahnemann read medicine and graduated from the University of Erlangen in 1775. Samuel Hahnemann soon became disillusioned with the medical practices of the time and set about to discover a

form of medicine that would be safe, gentle and effective. Through research over a number of years and with the help of friends and followers Hahnemann established the system of Homoeopathic Medicine as it is practised today. He died in Paris in 1843 in his late eighties.

MATERIA
MEDICA

A detailed list of homoeopathic remedies, in alphabetical order. These books give the sources of remedies and the symptom picture related to each one. This information is then used to match the symptoms of the patient with those of a medicine.

MEDICINE
PICTURES

A summary of symptoms that a substance is capable of producing in a healthy person and is therefore appropriate for the treatment of those symptoms.

MODALITIES

A term applied when the patient feels better or worse. For example heat, lying down, sitting up, fresh air etc. It is Modalities together with the medicine picture which results in the individual being treated rather than the illness.

MOTHER
TINCTURE

The starting material for the preparation of homoeopathic medicines denoted by the symbol O.

ORGANON

First published in 1810 and entitled *The Organon of Rational Healing*, this book is considered to be the most important of all Samuel Hahnemann's works, in which he has set out the whole of his philosophy on Homoeopathy.

POLYCRESTS

A medicine of value as a remedy for several conditions or diseases.

POTENCY

Dr Samuel Hahnemann discovered that the greater the dilution, the more potent the remedy became, therefore a Potency is the strength, or dilution, of a remedy.

PROVINGS

The name given to the systematic testing, by healthy people, of a potential homoeopathic medicine. The purpose of this was to catalogue all the symptoms induced by the substance, experienced by the person taking it. In this way Hahnemann and his followers established many homoeopathic remedies.

SIMILIA SIMILIBUS CURENTUR	The Law of Similars – 'Let like be treated by like'.
SUCCUSSION	Violent shaking, with impact, which takes place at each stage of sequential dilution when preparing a homoeopathic remedy.
TRITURATION	The method of producing a homoeopathic remedy from a substance which is insoluble. The substance is finely ground and mixed with an appropriate diluent.

Organisations

BLACKIE FOUNDATION TRUST

Established in 1971 by Dr Margery Blackie (then Homoeopathic Physician to HM the Queen), the Foundation aims to encourage study and education in the science of Homoeopathy. The Foundation also carries out and publishes the results of research.

The Blackie Foundation Trust
c/o 1 Upper Wimpole Street
London W1M 7TD

THE BRITISH ASSOCIATION OF HOMOEOPATHIC CHIROPODISTS

Founded by M Taufiq Khan MChS LCh SRCh MRIPHH, in 1978, this Association is a professional body open only to qualified chiropodists who are interested in learning Homoeopathic medicine and its use in conjunction with their own form of treatment.

The British Association of Homoeopathic Chiropodists
134 Montrose Avenue
Edgware
Middlesex HA8 0DR

Telephone: 081-959 5421

THE BRITISH ASSOCIATION OF HOMOEOPATHIC VETERINARY SURGEONS

Established in 1981 through the initiative of George MacLeod, the Association represents veterinary surgeons who are interested in, or who are practising Homoeopathy.

The Secretary
The British Association of Homoeopathic Veterinary Surgeons
Chinham House
Stanford-in-the-Vale
Nr Faringdon
Oxon SN7 8NQ

THE BRITISH HOMOEOPATHIC ASSOCIATION

Founded in 1902 and a registered charity. The Association has a membership open to professional people but exists primarily for the layman. The British Homoeopathic Association aims to spread the knowledge and use of homoeopathy and encourages the study of 'First Aid & Self Help Through Homoeopathy'. It holds regular meetings and publishes a bi-monthly Journal 'Homoeopathy' which is circulated to all members. There is also a library reserved for members. Supplies lists of doctors and vets who practise homoeopathy. Please send S.A.E.

The British Homoeopathic Association
27a Devonshire Street
London W1N 1RJ

Telephone: 071-935 2163

BRITISH HOMOEOPATHIC DENTAL ASSOCIATION

Because of the ever growing interest of dental surgeons in homoeopathy, the Faculty of Homoeopathy now holds special courses for dentists and the BHDA was formed in 1990.

British Homoeopathic Dental Association
Secretary: Miss C Price, BDS
12 Wellington Road
Watford
Herts

THE FACULTY OF HOMOEOPATHY

In 1844 Dr Frederick Harvey Foster Quin founded the British Homoeopathic Society. In 1943 this became the Faculty of Homoeopathy. The Faculty arranges Post-Graduate courses in homoeopathic medicine for doctors, veterinary surgeons, dental surgeons and pharmacists. Doctors can go on to become full members of the Faculty whilst Associate membership is offered to dentists, vets and pharmacists. The Faculty also publishes a quarterly Journal – The British Homoeopathic Journal.

The Faculty of Homoeopathy
The Royal London Homoeopathic Hospital
Great Ormond Street
London WC1N 3HR

Telephone: 071-837 8833 (Ask for the Faculty)

THE HAHNEMANN SOCIETY

Founded in 1958 by Dr Alva Benjamin. The objectives of this society are to educate the public in the principles of homoeopathy and in its safety and efficacy when treating both people and animals. Holds meetings, and an AGM with invited speakers, films and Self-Help Seminars. The Society also publishes a quarterly magazine, Health & Homoeopathy which is free to all members.

The Hahnemann Society
Hahnemann House
2 Powis Place
Great Ormond Street
London WC1N 3HR

Telephone: 071-837 3297

HOMOEOPATHIC PHARMACISTS ASSOCIATION

(Founded 1988)
92 Camden Road
Tunbridge Wells
Kent TN1 2QP

THE HOMOEOPATHIC TRUST FOR RESEARCH AND EDUCATION

A registered charity which promotes the advancement of Homoeopathy. Funds come entirely from donations, legacies and private contributions. It works in close co-operation with the Faculty.

The Homoeopathic Trust for Research and Education
Hahnemann House
2 Powis Place
Great Ormond Street
London WC1N 3HR

Telephone: 071-837 9469

THE NATIONAL ASSOCIATION OF HOMOEOPATHIC GROUPS

Founded in 1983 at the Faculty of Homoeopathy, the objectives of the Association are to co-ordinate the work of local Homoeopathic Groups and to liaise with the major homoeopathic, professional and Government bodies and with the general public. Their goal is the widespread availability of Homoeopathy under the National Health Service. New Homoeopathic Groups are invited to join the Association and should contact the Secretary.

Alma Cottage
Brainsmead
Cuckfield
West Sussex   RH17 5EY

THE SCOTTISH HOMOEOPATHIC RESEARCH AND EDUCATIONAL TRUST

The Trust gives financial assistance to doctors wishing to learn about Homoeopathy, or to qualify in the practice of Homoeopathy. It assists the Faculty with teaching and library services. It also helps to finance a Research Fellowship seeking confirmation of the action of homoeopathic remedies.

The Secretary
The Royal Bank of Scotland plc
30 Bothwell Street
Glasgow G2 6PB

THE SOCIETY OF HOMOEOPATHS

Founded in 1978 to meet the needs of those non-medical homoeopaths in this country and overseas who practise according to the principles established by Samuel Hahnemann. The Society has established a set of registration standards. Professional Homoeopaths who practise according to these standards are listed on the Society's Register. The Society also publishes a quarterly Journal 'The Homoeopath'.

2 Artizan Road
Northampton
NN1 4HU

Telephone: 0604 21400

LICENSED HOMOEOPATHIC MANUFACTURERS

A NELSON & CO LTD
Manufacturing Laboratories:

5 Endeavour Way
Wimbledon
London SW19 9UH

Telephone: 081 946 8527
Telex: 25774 Nelson G

WELEDA (UK) LTD
Heanor Road
Ilkeston
Derbyshire DE7 8DR

Telephone: 0602 303151

SPECIALIST HOMOEOPATHIC PHARMACIES
For a list of specialist homoeopathic pharmacies please contact the
British Homoeopathic Association at

27a Devonshire St
London W1N 1RJ

Telephone: 071-935 2163

Homoeopathic Hospitals and Clinics

THE BRISTOL HOMOEOPATHIC HOSPITAL
Homoeopathic medicine in Bristol began in 1852 with the establishment of a Dispensary in Queen Square. In 1883 a Homoeopathic Hospital was founded at 7 Brunswick Square and the adjoining Pembroke Cottage was purchased for use as a dispensary.

In 1948 the hospital came under the South West Regional Board and in 1964 was transferred to the United Bristol Hospitals Group. It is now part of the Bristol and Weston Health Authority and was the venue for the British Homoeopathic Congresses in 1954 and 1977.

GLASGOW HOMOEOPATHIC HOSPITAL
From a dispensary which was set up by a group of homoeopathic physicians in 1880 three institutions have developed, the major unit being the Glasgow Homoeopathic Hospital. The first homoeopathic hospital was established in 1914 in Lynedoch Crescent and was called the Houldsworth Hospital after a benefactor of that name. Its rapid growth led to the establishment of the present hospital in Great Western Road. Intensive courses are held every six months for general practitioners who wish to learn more about homoeopathy, or to prepare for the Faculty of Homoeopathy examinations.

The Glasgow Homoeopathic Hospital for Children was closed at the end of November 1979.

Glasgow Homoeopathic Hospital
1000 Great Western Road
Glasgow G12 0NR
Telephone: 041 339 0382

Glasgow Homoeopathic Out-Patient Department
Baillieston Health Institute
62 Buchanan Street
Baillieston
Glasgow G69
Telephone: 041 771 4490

Open mornings 9.30am Monday – Friday
                1.30pm Tuesday
Open evenings 5pm Monday and Wednesday
Telephone: 041 771 7396 and 041 771 7397

LIVERPOOL HOMOEOPATHIC CLINIC

The original Liverpool Homoeopathic Dispensary comprised the
South End Dispensary established in 1841, and the North End Dispensary, established in 1866 in response to an outbreak of cholera in
that year. The latter transferred to the Hahnemann Hospital when it
was built in Hope Street in 1887 and was then named the Liverpool
Hahnemann Hospital and Dispensary. The hospital came under State
control in 1948 under the National Health Service Act.

As a result of reorganisation on Merseyside it was decided to close
the hospital in April 1976. A Department of Homoeopathic Medicine
was then set up at the Liverpool Clinic in Myrtle Street with several
of the original hospital's staff; this was closed in 1980. Facilities are
now available at the Mossley Hill Hospital for out-patients, and a ten
bedded ward for in-patients.

Out-Patients Department
The Department of Homoeopathic Medicine
The Mossley Hill Hospital
Park Road
Liverpool L18
Telephone: 051 724 2335

MANCHESTER HOMOEOPATHIC CLINIC

The original homoeopathic dispensary in Manchester was founded in
Lower Byron Street in 1860. It was moved to new premises in

Jackson Street in 1887 and was named the Manchester Homoeopathic Institute and Dispensary. A new clinic was opened in Oxford Street by Sir John Weir in 1939 with Dr I. M. Burns as Senior Physician.

The old building was demolished in 1968 and the new modern clinic in Brunswick Street was opened in August 1971.

Manchester Homoeopathic Clinic
Brunswick Street
Manchester M13 9ST
Telephone: 061 273 2446

Clinic Hours: Monday – Friday, 9 – 10am and 5 – 6pm except Wednesday evening.

THE ROYAL LONDON HOMOEOPATHIC HOSPITAL
Patron: Her Majesty Queen Elizabeth II
The London Homoeopathic Hospital was founded by Dr Frederick F. H. Quin in 1849, twenty-one years after he had introduced homoeopathy into England. The hospital received the honour of Royal Patronage in 1920, when HRH the Duke of York became Patron and on his acceptance of the Presidency in 1924, was succeeded in the former office by HRH The Prince of Wales. Following the accession to the Throne of HRH Duke of York in 1936, the hospital was honoured by the Patronage of HM King George VI, which was conferred in February 1937. The Royal Charter of Incorporation was granted to the hospital by Privy Council on 19th December 1928.

It is also the registered address of the Faculty of Homoeopathy and is the principal centre in the United Kingdom for affording systematic instruction to Post-Graduates and qualified Practitioners in the principles and practice of Homoeopathy under the financial support of the Homoeopathic Research & Educational Trust.

Under the National Health Service Reorganisation Act 1973, the hospital no longer had an independent Management Committee and became administered by a District Management Team of the Camden & Islington Health Authority (Teaching) and now comes under Bloomsbury Health Authority as part of the North East Thames Regional Health Authority. In 1979 plans by the local area health authority to curtail severely the work of the hospital led to a petition containing 116,848 signatures being raised and a mass lobby of Parliament.

The Royal London Homoeopathic Hospital
Great Ormond Street
London WC1N 3HR
Telephone: 071-837 8833.
071-837 7821 (Out-Patients and Appointments)

TUNBRIDGE WELLS HOMOEOPATHIC HOSPITAL

Originally a dispensary, established in 1863, it transferred to another part of the town in 1866. The present small hospital was opened in Church Road and extensions were added in 1921 and 1930.

Tunbridge Wells Homoeopathic Hospital
Church Road
Tunbridge Wells
Kent
Telephone: 0892 542977

MID-CHESHIRE HOMOEOPATHIC CLINIC

Danebridge Medical Centre
Northwich
Cheshire CW9 5HR
Telephone: Northwich (0606) 49145

MARIGOLD TREATMENT CENTRES

Since 1975 Mr Khan has pioneered the use of external homoeopathic preparations in conjunction with Chiropodial Treatment. He discovered in 1979 that the Marigold (*Tagetes Sp*) is an effective remedy for skin, joints and nail conditions. Clinical research has shown that the success of *Tagetes Sp* is due to the combined effects of Chiropodial techniques and homoeopathic medicinal plant preparations, if used in accordance with homoeopathic principles.

Edgware, Middx. 081-959 5421

Hale Clinic, 7 Park Crescent
Telephone: 071-631 0156
London WC1. Telephone: 071-831 2962

International Organisations

AMERICAN FOUNDATION FOR HOMEOPATHY
1508 S Garfield
Alhambra
CA 91801 USA

NATIONAL CENTER FOR HOMOEOPATHY
801 N. Fairfax Street
Suite 306, Alexandria
Virginia 22314, USA
Telephone: (703) 548 7790

AUSTRALIAN FEDERATION OF HOMOEOPATHS INC
21 Bulah Close
Berowra Heights
Sydney NSW 2082 (02) 456-3602

HOMEOPATHIC EDUCATIONAL SERVICES
2124 Kittredge Street
Berkeley
CA 94704 USA

LIGA MEDICORUM HOMEOPATHICA INTERNATIONALIS
1068 21025 Dijon Cedex
FRANCE

NEW ZEALAND HOMOEOPATHIC SOCIETY
PO 67095, Mount Eden
Auckland
NEW ZEALAND

Recommended Reading

FOR BEGINNERS

HOMOEOPATHY FOR THE FAMILY
Probably the best selling introductory guide to the use of Homoeo-
pathic medicines in the home.
Wigmore Publications Ltd.

BEFORE THE DOCTOR COMES
Donovan Cox and Hyne Jones
Thorsons

THORSONS INTRODUCTORY GUIDE TO HOMOEOPATHY
Dr Anne Clover
A book designed for the non-medical reader. Supplying an outline of
the principles of Homoeopathy and how they can be applied today.
Thorsons

FIRST AID IN ACCIDENTS AND AILMENTS — Dr D. M. Gibson
The British Homoeopathic Association

FURTHER READING

THE PRESCRIBER
Dr J H Clarke
This best selling book enables anyone without a great knowledge of
homoeopathy to select a remedy most likely to be called for in a vast
number of ailments.
C W Daniels

MAGIC OF THE MINIMUM DOSE
Dr Dorothy Shepherd
C W Daniels

ADVANCED STUDY

HOMOEOPATHIC DRUG PICTURES
Dr M Tyler
A book which deals with 125 leading homoeopathic remedies.
C W Daniels

HOMOEOPATHIC MATERIA MEDICA, WITH REPERTORY
Dr W Boericke
Homoeopathic Book Service

AN INTRODUCTION TO HOMOEOPATHIC MEDICINE, 2nd Edition
Dr Hamish Boyd
A systematic introduction to homoeopathic medicine, setting out the basic philosophy and principles on which Homoeopathy is based. Containing practical information on case-taking, diagnosis and the application of remedies. Recommended for those wishing to make a study of this subject.
Beaconsfield

AN INTRODUCTION TO THE PRINCIPLES AND PRACTICE OF HOMO-EOPATHY
Dr C Wheeler
C W Daniels

VETERINARY HOMOEOPATHY

HOMOEOPATHY FOR PETS
Mr George Macleod, MREVS, DVSM
A simple and easy-to-use guide to the use of widely available homoeopathic remedies.
Homoeopathic Development Foundation Ltd

HOMOEOPATHIC FIRST-AID TREATMENT FOR PETS
Mr Francis Hunter, MRCVS
Thorsons

DOGS: HOMOEOPATHIC REMEDIES
Mr George Macleod, MRCVS, DVSM
A detailed work, by a world recognised authority on veterinary homoeopathy. Suitable for vets, breeders and owners.
C W Daniels

HOMOEOPATHIC TREATMENT OF SMALL ANIMALS
Mr C E I Day, MA, VetMB, MRCVS
A comprehensive survey of the principles and practice of homoeo-
pathy in the treatment of small animals. Invaluable for both vet
and owner.
C W Daniels

TREATMENT OF CATTLE BY HOMOEOPATHY
Mr George Macleod, MRCVS, DVSM
C W Daniels

TREATMENT OF HORSES BY HOMOEOPATHY
Mr George Macleod, MRCVS, DVSM
C W Daniels

CATS: HOMOEOPATHIC REMEDIES
Mr George Macleod, MRCVS, DVSM
C W Daniels

GOATS: HOMOEOPATHIC REMEDIES
Mr George Macleod, MRCVS, DVSM
C W Daniels

Publishers or Organisations Who Provide Information on Homoeopathy

BEACONSFIELD PUBLISHERS LTD
20 Chiltern Hills Road
Beaconsfield
Bucks HP9 1LP
Telephone: 0493 672118

BRITISH HOMOEOPATHIC ASSOCIATION
27a Devonshire Street
London W1N 1RJ
Telephone: 071-935 2163

C. W. DANIELS
1 Church Path
Saffron Walden
Essex CB10 1JP
Telephone: 0799 21909

INSIGHT EDITIONS
14 Longlands Glade
Worthing
Sussex BN14 9NR
Telephone: 0903 207011

THORSONS
A Division of HarperCollins*Publishers*
77-85 Fulham Palace Road
Hammersmith
London W6 8JB
Telephone: 081-741 7070

WIGMORE PUBLICATIONS LTD
10 Church Street
Steeple Bumpstead
Haverhill
Suffolk CB9 7DG
Telephone: 0440 730901

Index

Index

Of further interest . . .

HOMOEOPATHIC FIRST AID

Dr Anne Clover

Homoeopathic remedies can be used safely to help with many everyday ailments and emergencies. Using just 20 medicines you can give effective first-aid treatment for:

★ minior injuries
★ childhood illnesses
★ coughs, colds and other winter ailments
★ problems on holiday — travel sickness, diarrhoea etc
★ other family health problems

Dr Anne Clover also includes a short introduction to the principles and practice of homoeopathy. Here is a book no family medicine cabinet should be without.

THE HEALING POWER OF HERBAL TEAS

Ceres

This book will help you to discover the enormous potential of herbal teas and lotions. If, like many people today, you are becoming dissatisfied with relying on drugs for every minor ailment, why not turn instead to safer, non-habit-forming remedies like Chamomile, Caraway or Thyme teas. Herbal teas can help you to slim or to give up smoking; they can cheer you up or promote relaxation and restful sleep.

Ceres will show you how to plan and propagate a herb garden — either in the garden in herb beds, tubs and window boxes, or indoors on the kitchen window sill — and she gives advice about drying and preserving herbs for future use. Each herb is then fully described, with information on its therapeutic purpose and the best method of using it — in tisane, infusion or lotion form. As well as the alphabetical sections on the herbs themselves, there is also a therapeutic index to help you to find those herbs most beneficial in dealing with specific common ailments.

THORSONS INTRODUCTORY GUIDE TO HOMOEOPATHY

Dr Anne Clover

Homoeopathy is a remarkable system of medicine founded by Samuel Hahnemann, a German physician, nearly two hundred years ago, which is enjoying a widespread revival of interest. The basis of homoeopathy is treating likes with likes, but there is a lot more to it than that.

Dr Anne Clover, a medically trained doctor who practises homoeopathy and is a hospital consultant in homoeopathic medicine, outlines Hahnemann's original discoveries and describes in easy to read style all about homoeopathy today and how it can help you.

An invaluable guide for those coming into contact with homoeopathic medicine for the first time, and a useful and fascinating book for all.

HOMOEOPATHIC FIRST AID	0 7225 2107 3	£4.99 ☐
THE HEALING POWER OF HERBAL TEAS	0 7225 1575 8	£3.99 ☐
THORSONS INTRODUCTORY GUIDE TO HOMOEOPATHY	0 7225 2529 X	£3.99 ☐
THORSONS INTRODUCTORY GUIDE TO ACUPUNCTURE	0 7225 2531 1	£3.99 ☐
THORSONS INTRODUCTORY GUIDE TO CHIROPRACTIC	0 7225 2526 5	£3.99 ☐
THORSONS INTRODUCTORY GUIDE TO IRIDOLOGY	0 7225 2530 3	£3.99 ☐
THORSONS INTRODUCTORY GUIDE TO OSTEOPATHY	0 7225 2532 X	£3.99 ☐
THORSONS INTRODUCTORY GUIDE TO REFLEXOLOGY	0 7225 2528 1	£3.99 ☐

All these books are available at your local bookseller or can be ordered direct from the publishers.

To order direct just tick the titles you want and fill in the form below:

Name: _____

Address: _____

_____

_____ Postcode: _____

Send to: Thorsons Mail Order, Dept 3L, HarperCollins*Publishers*, Westerhill Road, Bishopbriggs, Glasgow G64 2QT.
Please enclose a cheque or postal order or debit my Visa/Access account —

Credit card no: ☐☐☐☐☐☐☐☐☐☐☐☐☐☐☐☐☐

Expiry date: _____

Signature: _____

— to the value of the cover price plus:
UK & BFPO: Add £1.00 for the first book and 25p for each additional book ordered.
Overseas orders including Eire: Please add £2.95 service charge. Books will be sent by surface mail but quotes for airmail despatches will be given on request.

24 HOUR TELEPHONE . ORDERING SERVICE FOR ACCESS/VISA CARDHOLDERS — TEL: 041 772 2281.